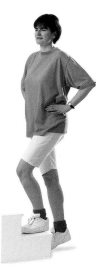

HEALTH AND HEALING
THE NATURAL WAY

DIET AND
WEIGHT CONTROL

Reader's
Digest

PUBLISHED BY

THE READER'S DIGEST ASSOCIATION LIMITED

LONDON NEW YORK MONTREAL SYDNEY CAPE TOWN

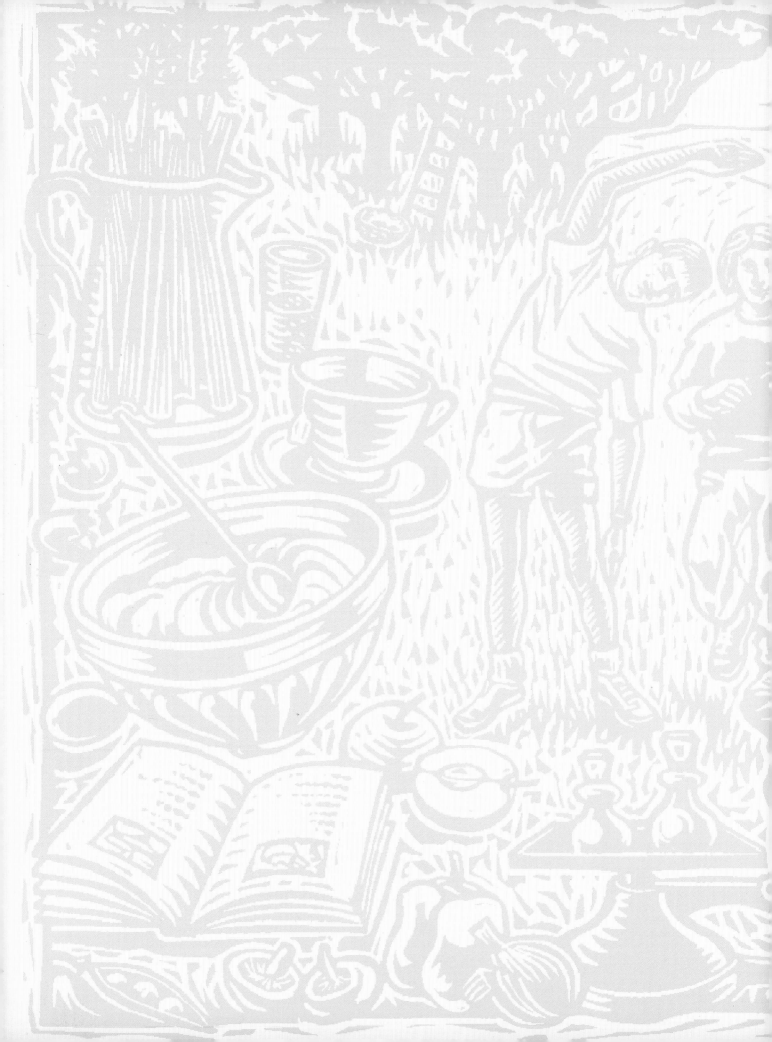

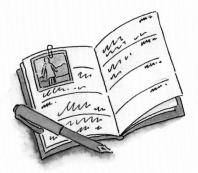

HEALTH AND HEALING
THE NATURAL WAY

DIET AND WEIGHT CONTROL

PUBLISHED BY

THE READER'S DIGEST ASSOCIATION, INC.

PLEASANTVILLE, NEW YORK / MONTREAL

A Reader's Digest Book
Produced by
Carroll & Brown Limited, London

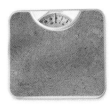

CARROLL & BROWN

Publishing Director Denis Kennedy
Art Director Chrissie Lloyd

Managing Editor Sandra Rigby

Editor Joanne Stanford
Assistant Editor Joel Levy

Art Editor Gilda Pacitti
Designer Jonathan Wainwright

Photographers Jules Selmes, David Murray

Production Christine Corton, Wendy Rogers

Computer Management John Clifford

First English Edition Copyright © 1997
The Reader's Digest Association Limited,
11 Westferry Circus, Canary Wharf,
London E14 4HE

Reprinted with amendments 1998

CONSULTANT

Dr. Susan Jebb BSc, SRD, PhD
Head of Obesity Research, MRC Dunn Nutrition Centre

CONTRIBUTORS

Shirley Bond SRD
State registered dietitian and home economist

Tamsin Burnett-Hall
Home economist

Gary Frost BSc, SRD
State registered dietitian

Roger Newman-Turner BAc, ND, DO, MRO, MRN
Registered naturopath, osteopath and acupuncturist

Maria Pufulete
BSc Food Science

Claire Potter AFAA
Lifestyle planning and health and fitness consultant

Nicola Seabrook BSc, SRD
State registered dietitian

Carolyn Summerbell BSc, SRD
State registered dietitian

Nick Troop BSc, DHP
Psychologist in eating disorders

FOR READER'S DIGEST

Project Editor Gayla Visalli

READER'S DIGEST GENERAL BOOKS

Editor in Chief, U.S. General Books Chris Cavanaugh
Editorial Director, health & medicine Wayne Kalyn
Design Director, health & medicine Barbara Rietschel

The information in this book is for reference only;
it is not intended as a substitute for a doctor's diagnosis and care.
The editors urge anyone with continuing medical problems
or symptoms to consult a doctor.

DIET AND WEIGHT CONTROL

More and more people today are choosing to take greater responsibility for their own health rather than relying on their doctor to step in with a cure when something goes wrong. We now recognize that we can influence our health by making certain improvements in lifestyle—eating better, doing more exercise, and taking measures to reduce stress. People are also becoming increasingly aware that there are other healing methods— some new, others ancient—that can help prevent illness or be used as complements to orthodox medicine.

The series *Health and Healing the Natural Way* can help you make your own health choices by giving you clear, comprehensive, straightforward, and encouraging information and advice about methods of improving your health. The series explains the many different natural therapies now available, including aromatherapy, herbalism, acupressure, and a number of others, as well as the circumstances in which they benefit you when used in conjunction with conventional medicine.

The approach of *DIET AND WEIGHT CONTROL* is to emphasize that, despite the ever-growing dieting industry, with its gimmicks, aids, and miracle diets, there really is no replacement for eating the correct balance of the right foods and living an active life. The book dispels many of the dieting myths and misleading messages about ideal body shape espoused by the media. It tells you how to determine what is truly a healthy body weight and reveals the factors, both physical and psychological, that influence your weight. You will find all the information necessary for you to assess your current weight, plus practical advice on how to take charge of your eating habits. If you are overweight or underweight for your height, setting a sensible weight target, reaching it, and maintaining it will lower your risks for disorders such as diabetes and coronary heart disease and increase your general health and well-being.

CONTENTS

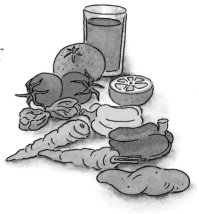

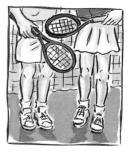

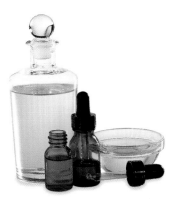
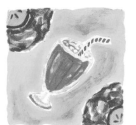

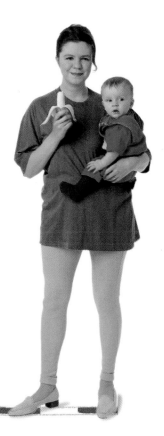
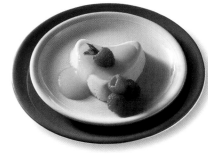

THE TRUTH ABOUT WEIGHT CONTROL

Effective weight management involves more than short-term fads: it is about making permanent changes to your eating habits and lifestyle.

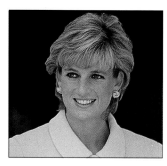

DIANA, PRINCESS OF WALES
Diana was known to have suffered from the chronic eating disorder, bulimia. Her success in overcoming bulimia has given hope to other sufferers.

Even though Western society is becoming increasingly concerned about weight control, much evidence points to the fact that we are far from successful at managing our weight. At one end of the spectrum eating disorders such as anorexia and bulimia are becoming more prevalent. At the other end, being overweight is the most prevalent nutrition-related health problem. About 50 percent of adults in the United States are overweight and of these, about 30 percent are obese, defined as being 20 percent or more above desirable weight. Particularly worrying is the fact that obesity is increasing among children. Why is effective weight control such a problem today? And why do so many people find it so hard to achieve and maintain a healthy weight?

OUR MODERN LIFESTYLE

The answer lies in the changes in lifestyle and types of food that have become available in Western countries over the past 60 years. Modern technology has reduced the amount of physical activity in our daily lives at every level, from transportation to labor-saving devices in the home and at work. The automobile has had a dramatic effect on the average person's daily activity levels: even walking at a moderate pace burns 250 calories an hour, whereas driving burns only 100 calories. At the same time, because of changes in social and work habits, mealtimes are less structured. On a regular basis, many people buy ready-made meals from a supermarket or take-out foods from a delicatessen, which are often high in fat. And these are supplemented frequently with high-calorie snacks. A recent study revealed that up to 45 per cent of the average child's energy intake comes from snacks rather than regular meals. This combination of high-fat foods and increasingly sedentary lives is the principal reason for the steady weight gain recorded in North American countries since the Second

BE REALISTIC!
Some people let the bathroom scales rule their life, looking almost daily for proof of weight reduction. Shedding pounds too quickly, however, is not healthy; a good weight-loss plan should advocate a weight loss of only 0.5–1 kg (1-2 lbs) a week.

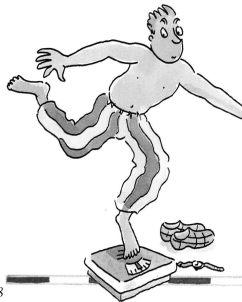

World War. The argument that lifestyle is primarily to blame is supported by the experience of immigrants from less wealthy countries who have moved to the affluent West. After a comparatively short time immigrant populations adopting the Western lifestyle exhibit similar diet-related problems, including obesity, to those in their adoptive countries.

A more fundamental problem with weight control is inherent in basic human physiology. Our bodies are well designed to help us deal with starvation. In fact, as we eat less our bodies become more and more efficient at functioning on less food. The metabolism slows down and we become more lethargic in order to conserve energy. This is why it is hard to continue losing weight by dieting alone: the body adapts to the change in energy intake and simply slows down all nonessential functions. The reason is that physiologically we are still hunter-gatherers like our Stone Age ancestors. Our bodies are prepared for periods of semistarvation, but when food is plentiful we are happy to eat more, even if we are not physically in need of food. During the Stone Age, however, people led far more physical lives. Constantly on the move and actively engaged in searching for food, they had energy needs higher than those of the average desk worker today. In fact anthropologists draw direct correlations between the level of development of a society (with Stone Age societies at one end of the spectrum and industrialized ones at the other) and the weight-related diseases and disorders from which it suffers. Diet and lifestyle underlie this correlation.

SO HOW DO YOU CONTROL WEIGHT?

Research has shown that in order to control weight properly we need to balance energy intake and energy expenditure in our daily lives. In other words, we have to make sure that we are eating the right amount of food for the amount of activity we perform daily. Our energy requirements are governed by a number of factors. To a large extent gender determines our fuel requirements: men tend to need more food than women because a greater percentage of their body is muscle, and muscle burns more energy. Calorie requirements also change throughout our lives: children need more energy to support their growth, while adults need less as they grow older. Then there are exceptional cases: athletes need more food than average people to sustain their high energy output. An athlete may burn in excess of 4,000 calories a day, whereas a sedentary man

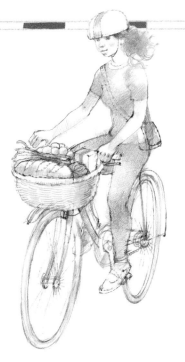

THE ROAD TO SUCCESS
Combining regular exercise and a healthy diet is the way to lose weight most successfully. Exercise can be increased in simple ways, for example, by walking or cycling when you would normally use the car.

NATHAN PRITIKIN
The Pritikin diet, one of the most popular in recent years, was devised by Nathan Pritikin in the 1970s (see page 108). Most nutritionists today, however, argue that his diet is too restrictive to be practical. Long-term weight control requires sustainable dietary changes.

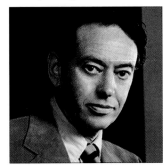

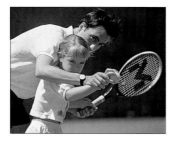

A HEALTHY START TO LIFE
It is important to encourage children to enjoy exercise by nurturing any interest they show in a particular sport.

needs only about 2,200 calories a day. With any increase in activity the body burns more calories. Furthermore, regular sustained exercise can raise the metabolic rate, meaning that the body uses more energy in every activity, from breathing to eating to sleeping to participating in sports.

It is also important to look at the type of food being consumed. Weight control isn't simply about restricting calorie intake, it's about getting the right balance of foods in the diet. The good news here is that eating healthfully by reducing fat and eating more complex carbohydrates (starches), especially in whole-grain forms, plus more fruits and vegetables, is also a successful plan for weight control. Research has shown that complex carbohydrates are the body's preferred source of energy. Dietary fat, on the other hand, tends to be simply stored by the body.

ARE THERE ANY SHORTCUTS?

A dramatic reduction in calories can often produce rapid weight loss. Many people sign up for a variety of programs and classes, often based on meal substitutes, to get results in just weeks. But the vast majority of people who lose weight in this way simply regain it over the following months. People who make a habit of shortcut dieting—whose weight is constantly "yo-yoing"—may be doing themselves more harm than good, both physically and mentally. For example, dieters who quickly regain all the weight they have lost often feel guilty and depressed by their failure to keep to the diet.

HOME-GROWN GOODNESS
Growing your own fruits and vegetables will ensure that you always have something fresh and flavorsome for the table. It can save money, give you great satisfaction, and also be good exercise.

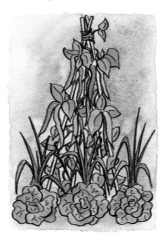

Other people turn to clinics that offer cosmetic surgery or drug treatment. A variety of cosmetic procedures are available, from liposuction to surgical intervention in the gut, the latter designed to prevent or reduce eating or inhibit the digestion or absorption of food. The drugs used may have side effects and can currently be prescribed for just a limited period of time. Such treatments are extreme and recommended only for people whose health is in immediate danger because of a weight problem.

The potential market for a drug that would cure obesity and reduce anyone's weight is huge, and pharmaceutical companies invest heavily in research into the biology of eating, appetite, and weight control. But despite many exciting discoveries, from the role of hormones to the discovery of a gene that appears to control obesity in mice (the *ob* gene), the overwhelming message to emerge from research is that the causes of human weight problems are too complex to be isolated to a single factor. This means that there is not, and is unlikely to be, a "magic pill" that can be taken to help us banish fat and shed weight without any conscious effort.

Nutritionists agree that the only truly successful way to lose weight is through changes in diet and activity, an approach that takes into account your whole lifestyle. The benefits can include more energy, better sleep, and a range of improvements to general well-being, from lower blood pressure to enhanced self-confidence.

DO YOU NEED TO CHANGE YOUR WEIGHT?

Many people, particularly women, immediately answer yes to this question, but it is important to give the answer more careful thought. If you believe that you need to alter your weight, the first step is to accurately measure your weight in relation to your height and frame. The most respected method for doing this is the Body Mass Index, orBMI, system (see page 25). Establishing your BMI will tell you whether you are underweight, of average weight, overweight, or obese. You can then make a sensible decision about the degree to which you might need to make changes.

Knowing exactly why you want to diet is important if you are to set realistic goals for yourself. The best reason to lose weight is for your general health. Being obese (having a BMI of over 30) is a major risk factor for a variety of disorders, including heart disease, diabetes, and some cancers. Obesity can also have a detrimental effect on self-esteem and confidence, and many obese people suffer from depression.

But some persons who are overweight rather than obese, or who may even be of normal weight, see losing poundage as a way to solve many of the other things they are unhappy about in their lives. Problems at work or with partners or other family members can all be blamed on their excess weight. Weight loss cannot provide a magical solution to other problems, and if this is an underlying reason for wanting to lose weight, it is important to examine more closely the sources of unhappiness in your life. Dieting for reasons unrelated to actual weight is a serious risk factor for some eating disorders. Studies show that the instance of bulimia (see page 39), for example, tripled between 1988 and 1993. Anorexia nervosa is also on the rise. Many people, especially young women, are strongly influenced by the media and its obsession with slim models. Fashions change,

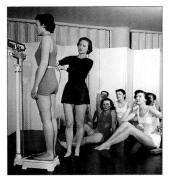

THE DIETING FASHION
Since the Second World War women have become increasingly obsessed about weight, often without cause. The above women, all within a healthy weight range for their age and height, are being persuaded to lose extra pounds during a three-week health and beauty course.

HERE'S TO YOUR HEALTH
A weight-loss diet should always be undertaken with care. Some strict diets are lacking in the vitamins and minerals that are essential for good health.

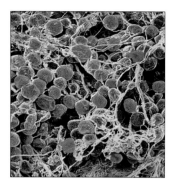

THE ROLE OF ADIPOSE
Fat cells, the brown and red rounded cells shown above, are held within adipose tissue in the body. Dietary fat that has not been burned off by the body is stored in these cells.

CUTTING BACK ON FAT
Trimming fat from chops and bacon before cooking them can significantly reduce your fat intake. Before serving meat, blot off excess fat with paper towels.

however, and women who in the 19th century were considered great beauties are seen today as significantly overweight. Part of effective weight control is about understanding the difference between healthy weight and fashionable weight, and distancing yourself from unrealistic goals dictated by society.

SUSTAINABLE WEIGHT CONTROL

Diet and Weight Control covers all of these issues, from first principles to practical tips. It discusses normal body shape and size, the factors that influence weight, and practices that can be adopted to manage and reduce weight.

Chapter 1 contrasts the pressures imposed by the media on people's self-image with the truth about what is a normal and healthy body shape. It explains how to tell if you are really overweight or underweight and if you need to take action. Chapter 2 discusses the physical and psychological factors that influence and determine your weight. Emerging discoveries in the fields of genetics, hormones, and pharmaceutical research are covered, together with the basic anatomy, physiology, and psychology of appetite and eating. Chapter 3 presents a general overview of how to manage weight, looking at why we eat too much or too little, and what we should eat to stay healthy throughout our lives. Chapter 4 explains the details of how different types of food affect weight.

Chapters 5, 6, and 7 cover, respectively, the theories and practices of exercise, natural therapies, and diet with regard to weight control. Each chapter discusses the elements involved and the practical steps you can take for yourself, including advice on how to involve your whole family, old and young. Chapter 8 presents a fully integrated personal weight-control plan that you can adapt to your own needs and goals, with tips on how to fit a healthy diet, one that fulfills the needs of both you and your family, into a busy schedule. Menus and recipes in Chapter 9 show you how to apply the principles of low-fat cooking to your own meal planning. Throughout the book special sections describe the roles of different professionals in the field of diet and weight control, while selected case studies illustrate common problems that can arise and how to deal with them. *DIET AND WEIGHT CONTROL* offers no crash diets or miracle methods. Instead it clearly sets out the basic tenets of achievable, sustainable weight control for a healthier, happier life.

How much do you know about weight control?

There are many misconceptions in the field of weight control and dieting. Even the simplest task of estimating exactly how much you eat during the day is difficult to do accurately. You may be surprised at just how much fat and sugar you consume from processed foods or unaware of the numerous health benefits that simple lifestyle changes, such as walking up the stairs instead of taking the elevator, can bring in the long term.

Q **WOULD YOU LIKE TO LOSE 5 kg (11 lb) IN TWO WEEKS?**
If you answered "yes," then you're probably making a serious mistake. Diet regimens that produce such dramatic effects usually make you eat a severely unbalanced diet, and the weight reduction you achieve is more from fluid and protein loss than from shedding fat. This is not a healthy approach, and the weight is likely to be quickly regained when you stop the diet and resume normal eating patterns. See Chapter 7.

Q **DO YOU FIND IT IMPOSSIBLE TO RESIST FATTY FOODS?**
Research shows that most people find fatty foods more tasty and filling than other types of foods. Some theorists argue that this reflects our Stone Age past: for our Neolithic ancestors fat was a rare and potentially life-saving treat. Today we have to work hard to overcome our evolutionary predisposition for fatty foods. *DIET AND WEIGHT CONTROL* provides a wealth of tips and food ideas, from snacks to full meals, to help you do just that. See Chapters 4 and 9.

Q **DO YOU LOOK AT FOOD LABELS?**
Many people don't check the calorie and fat content of the foods they purchase, and yet surprising discoveries can be made by doing this. Learning which foods are a healthy buy is an important part of a weight-control plan. Chapter 4 looks into the value of "health foods," shows you how to calculate the fat content of foods, and provides a calorie and fat content chart of some popular foods. The "cutting calories" boxes in every chapter will also help you make healthy food choices.

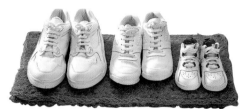

A FAMILY COMMITMENT
Every member of the family can benefit from increasing their level of exercise, and it is especially important for children in today's computer-game age. Make the outdoors fun for children by exercising as a family; playing football in the park and going on walks or bicycle rides all provide good aerobic activity.

SCHOOL LUNCHES
Encourage children to adopt healthy eating habits from an early age. Include fresh or dried fruit in their packed lunches rather than cookies or cake. Provide a treat once in a while, but remember that a sweet tooth gained at this age is likely to stay with them throughout adulthood.

Q DO YOU HAVE A SEDENTARY JOB?

Scientists link rising rates of obesity to two factors. One is the diet of modern society. The other is the steady decline in levels of physical activity. Automation and labor-saving devices allow many people to lead more sedentary lives, especially if they work in jobs where they sit all day. Even modest changes to your routine, like getting off the bus two stops from home and walking the rest of the way, can radically improve your activity levels. Every small change you make will help with losing weight and sustaining that reduction, while at the same time improving your health and well-being. Chapter 5 describes the ways in which you can bring exercise into your life. "Quick fitness tips" in every chapter offer easy-to-implement advice on increasing your day-to-day activity levels, while "burning off calories" boxes explain various forms of exercise and the muscle groups targeted by each one.

Q DO YOU FIND MOST LIFESTYLE ADVICE TOO UNREALISTIC TO ASPIRE TO?

Sweeping statements about the need to change your lifestyle and to replace your normal diet with one of bran and beans are not very helpful. Most people do not want to become vegetarians or fitness fanatics, while others may be concerned about the expense of organic foods and exercise classes. The personal weight-control plans in Chapter 8 will help you to set realistic goals. This chapter also offers advice on how to solve common lifestyle problems.

Q DOES YOUR FAMILY SABOTAGE YOUR HEALTHY EATING INTENTIONS?

Many people find that their families can make weight-control plans difficult to implement. Children, especially, can be fussy eaters and reject changes to healthful, low-fat foods. Chapter 3 looks at the different food requirements of children and adults and shows you how to ensure that children receive the right level of nutrition without compromising your own low-fat approach. The recipes in Chapter 9 will give you ideas on how to make family meals low in fat but high in flavor and nutrients. There are also some creative recipes that may help to persuade a reluctant partner that dietary changes not only make health sense but can also be delicious.

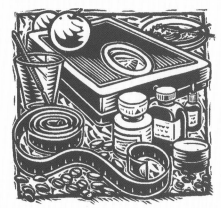

CHAPTER 1

IS YOUR WEIGHT HEALTHY?

*The decision to begin a weight-loss program
needs to be taken with care. Assessing the reasons
why you are unhappy with your weight, examining
your general health and well-being, and recognizing
a distinction between your own body shape
and unrealistic images promoted by society
are important first steps to take.*

HEALTHY WEIGHT

Ideal weight can be defined in two ways: in terms of attractiveness and in light of good health. The two definitions do not necessarily mean the same thing.

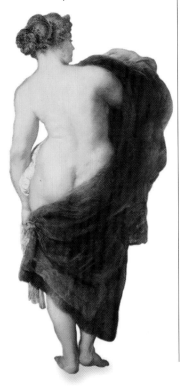

CHANGING TIMES
This detail taken from Rubens' Judgement of Paris *shows how much society's perception of human beauty has changed over the years. Today, this figure would be deemed too overweight to be fashionable.*

It is important to recognize the extent to which the perception of ideal weight is influenced by fashion, advertising, and the media. The images presented to society do not always represent healthy body-weight statistics, and they make it more difficult to set realistic weight goals. An attempt to attain an unrealistic body shape is bound to fail and may even be dangerous.

IMAGE AND WEIGHT
The ideal attractive body image changes over time and varies from one culture to another. In the West at present the favored shape is thin, and there has been a great deal of speculation as to why this should be so.

Since the 1950s there has been a marked increase in leisure time, travel, and outdoor pursuits. Many fashion commentators believe that activities such as swimming, tennis, and travel, once restricted to the privileged classes, have been responsible for promoting the slim look, as women strive to attain a figure suitable for public display at the beach, pool, or gym. Others argue that society has come to associate desirability with youth. The slim, adolescent figure has become the ideal, and models as young as 15 set the standards for the ideal figure. The fashion industry has been blamed for preferring their clothes to be modeled on very thin models. Designers argue back that clothes simply look better on a thin, broad-shouldered body type and that they are committed to marketing their designs in the most effective way possible.

Whatever the reasons behind society's fixation with slimness, the idea is reinforced in almost every aspect of daily life through advertising and the media. Images of flat-stomached, adolescent girls on billboards and buses and in magazines, television programs, and films, sell everything from jeans to elegant automobiles to dreamy vacations.

Subconsciously, we receive the message that being thin will make us more desirable, successful, and happy.

But fashions change. A look at Western art reveals that ideal female beauty used to be represented by significantly rounder women. Today, the Venus de Milo would be considered to have large thighs and be in need of tummy firming exercises. Rubens' nudes are even more voluptuous, and Renoir's women are uniformly plump. Even in this century, the standard female figure was once fuller (see box, opposite page).

WHAT IS NORMAL?
What was considered ideal body weight used to be derived from charts published by the American Metropolitan Life Insurance Company. The company calculated the lowest mortality associated with a particular weight for a given height, based on the medical records of the company's clients. From this data they drew up optimum weights for people of all heights, but these charts have changed significantly since they first appeared in the 1920s. It was realized that the original samples were unrepresentative, and optimum weights have gradually been increasing over the past few decades.

Today a respected method for assessing weight is the Body Mass Index, or BMI (see page 25), calculated by dividing your weight

DID YOU KNOW?
In many countries plumpness is still considered attractive. The Chinese associate a full figure with prosperity and longevity, and in many Arab countries it is symbolic of fertility and womanhood. In these cultures being plump not only symbolizes beauty but also conforms to the stereotype of the caring, reliable mother.

THE CHANGING IMAGE OF IDEAL BODY WEIGHT

The fashion industry's image of ideal body weight has changed dramatically through the years and is becoming increasingly unrealistic. For the majority of ordinary women, this perceived ideal shape is a physical impossibility.

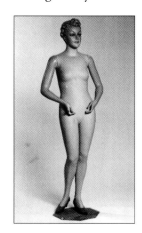

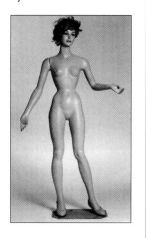

1930 VERSUS 1960
A study by the University Central Hospital in Helsinki, Finland, found that before the 1950s the percentage of body fat shown on mannequins was within a desirably healthy range. Since the 1950s, however, the models have gradually become too thin to be representative of a healthy weight. By 1960 (right) impossibly narrow waists and hips and thin thighs had replaced the more realistic pear-shape of the 1930s (left). Unfortunately, the 1960 figure is still in vogue today.

in kilograms by your height in meters squared. (To convert kilograms to pounds, multiply by 2.2046; to convert centimeters to inches, divide by 2.54.) Optimum BMIs are arrived at by measuring mortality against weight for height. Even though mortality risks vary from country to country, it is possible to say that the optimum BMI for both men and women is between 20 and 25. Individuals with a BMI greater than 30 are classified as obese and should lose weight for the benefit of their health.

If your BMI is within the appropriate range for your weight and height but you still want to improve your shape, exercises targeted to tone the particular part of the body you are unhappy with may be more worthwhile than trying to lose weight.

WEIGHT AND THE INDIVIDUAL

Optimum weight for an individual may vary over time. Physiological changes affect weight during a lifetime (see Chapter 2), and for women there are the added effects of the menstrual cycle, pregnancy, and menopause.

From birth to childhood

As there is little data on how weight gain during the early years of life relates to long-term health, it is difficult to give precise healthy weight figures for children. But it is important to monitor your child's growth and health so that you can identify when weight problems are sufficiently severe to warrant seeking medical advice. The chart on page 18 shows average growth rates from birth to adolescence. Since children differ in their genetic potential for growth, however, a group of normal children of the same age will vary in weight and height. But a normal child should not be greatly dissimilar to other children of the same age. If you are concerned, discuss it with your doctor.

With obese children, it is important to help them achieve a healthy balanced diet that maintains a constant weight. This will allow normal growth to continue, whereas more severe measures to produce weight loss can interfere with this process. As such children gain height, they should effectively grow into their weight.

From adolescence to adulthood

Weight and height increase at a steady rate throughout childhood until the onset of puberty, when there is a sudden growth spurt. Extra food is required at this time to fuel the development of muscle, bone, and other tissues. This spurt continues until the late teens, when bone growth slows down and a little extra muscle is put on, unless muscle building exercises are carried out.

Girls lay down extra fat in adolescence, which is distributed to help develop female characteristics like fuller breasts and rounded hips. Some adolescents put on extra weight due to a sedentary lifestyle; this may lead to a weight problem that lasts into adulthood, unless steps are taken to exercise regularly while following a healthy, balanced diet.

SOCIAL RULES
The fashion world's obsession with the super-slim figure has been directly linked to an increase in eating disorders seen in much of the developed world.

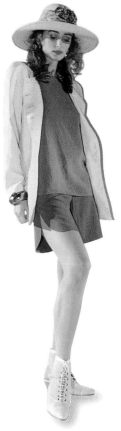

HEALTHY WEIGHT GAIN DURING PREGNANCY

During pregnancy you should put on some weight for the benefit of both yourself and the baby. The following figures are a guide to how much additional weight you should be aiming for, depending on your BMI (see page 25) at the baby's conception:

▶ *Underweight with a BMI below 19.8: 12.5–18 kg (28–40 lb)*

▶ *Normal weight with a BMI of 19.8–26: 11.5–16 kg (25–35 lb)*

▶ *Overweight with a BMI of 26–29: 7–11.5 kg (15–25 lb)*

▶ *Obese with a BMI over 30: at least 6 kg (13 lb)*

AVERAGE WEIGHTS FOR CHILDREN (lb)

This growth table helps you monitor and record the development of your child from baby to teenager. It shows the expected weight for healthy, average children and can alert you to possible irregularities at an early stage in their development.

AGE	Birth	6–12 m	1–2 y	3–4 y	5–6 y	7–8 y	9–10 y	11–12 y	13–14 y	15–16 y	17–18 y
BOYS	6.5–9	13	26	35	44	53	64	77	99	128	141
GIRLS	6.5–9	13	26	35	44	53	64	82	110	123	128

Pregnancy and breast-feeding

Pregnancy is a period of considerable metabolic and nutritional change. Many people naturally assume that a mother needs a lot of additional energy to meet the demands placed on her body by the rapid growth of her baby, the placenta, and other new tissues of pregnancy. But just how much a pregnant woman actually needs in extra energy intake is a matter for debate.

Recent studies have revealed that there is an extraordinary range in the way women's bodies respond to pregnancy. Some women lay down huge amounts of body fat, while others gain very little. Some experience a significant increase in their metabolic rate (see page 29) and therefore use more energy than before they became pregnant, while others develop a lower rate. These changes last only while the woman is pregnant and seem to be part of the body's way of sensing how well-nourished a woman is, and then responding by providing the best conditions for the growing baby.

During pregnancy, most women should eat as much or as little as their appetites tell them to, but should consult their doctors if they put on excessive weight or very little weight in relation to their body mass index number (see far left). Women who gain excessive weight are at higher risk of having complications during pregnancy and are more likely to retain the extra pounds afterward. In contrast, women who gain too little weight are at higher risk of having low-birth-weight or premature babies.

Women should not diet during pregnancy, because it can be dangerous. There is evidence that severe dieting may limit the growth of the baby and ultimately be responsible for an infant with low birth weight. Severe dieting during breastfeeding can also take a toll on a mother's health and may cause a decrease in milk production

EXERCISING SAFELY DURING PREGNANCY

Regular exercise during pregnancy will help you retain muscle tone and prevent build-up of fat. It can also contribute to a smooth, less painful birth. Devise an exercise program after consultation with your doctor and then set aside a set time, at least three times a week, to exercise. It's important to warm up before exercising by stretching all your muscles thoroughly, and take time to cool down and relax afterward.

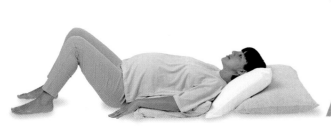

EXERCISING THE PELVIC FLOOR MUSCLES
These muscles cradle and protect the womb. Lie flat on your back with knees bent. Squeeze your pelvic muscles, as if to stop a flow of urine, and hold for 10 seconds; repeat 10 times.

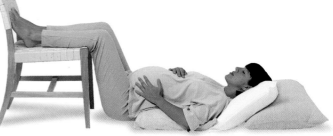

RELAXATION
Thoroughly relaxing after exercise is vital. Lying flat on your back with your legs raised on a bed or chair is especially relaxing and is particularly good for swollen ankles and feet.

THE MENOPAUSE AND WEIGHT GAIN

Women may experience slight weight gain after menopause. This is due in part to the slowing of metabolism, but mostly it is just a by-product of the aging process and a decrease in physical activity. More pronounced, however, is the change in fat distribution: after menopause, fat is deposited around the stomach. This occurs as a result of reduced levels of estrogen in the body.

FAT REDISTRIBUTION
Before menopause (left), fat is distributed around the buttocks and thighs as well as the shoulders and breasts. After menopause (right), fat tends to collect on the stomach, abdomen, and breasts.

Middle age

People tend to get fatter as they grow older, and many people complain of "middle-age spread." There is a small decline in the body's metabolic rate beginning at about age 30 (approximately 2 percent for each subsequent decade), but more significant is the marked decrease in physical activity that commonly occurs in this age group. Active participation in sports steadily declines with age, and more time is spent watching television or in other sedentary activities. If energy intake is not reduced in proportion to these changes, weight will be gained.

At the same time muscle cells become weaker (atrophy) and there is a shift in the body's overall ratio of muscle to fat; there tends to be more fatty tissue and less lean. Regular exercise helps slow down muscle atrophy and prevent the build up of fat, so it's necessary to maintain or even increase levels of physical activity as one grows older. This may mean having to find new activities that are easily fitted into daily routines. Walking 30 minutes each day, for example, can not only improve health but also help control weight.

Menopause

The question of whether or not menopause alters a woman's body weight remains a controversial one. While many women claim that they have put on weight after menopause, most studies demonstrate that this can be accounted for by the simple fact that people tend to gain weight as they get older anyway, suggesting that age and not the menopause is responsible for the increase. However, the menopause is associated with changes in fat distribution (see above). Some women who have been prescribed hormone replacement therapy, or HRT, to help relieve the symptoms of menopause believe that the treatment is the cause of their weight gain. While there is no conclusive evidence to support this claim, an increase in water retention, and therefore puffiness, is one of the potential side effects of HRT.

Old age

By the age of 70, many people's bodies have about twice as much fat as when they were in their 30s and only about half as much muscle tissue. Keeping active helps preserve

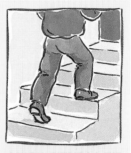

QUICK FITNESS TIP
Taking the stairs instead of the elevator will burn a few extra calories and tone your leg muscles.

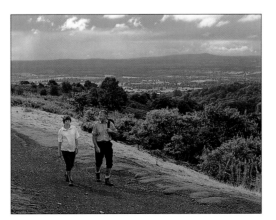

MAINTAINING FLEXIBILITY
Many older people suffer from joint problems as they become less active. Light aerobic exercise such as walking, ballroom dancing, or swimming can help prevent joints from becoming too stiff and will boost the body's energy expenditure.

muscle tissue and maintain a desirable weight, but being slightly overweight in old age is associated with only modest health risks. This is a time to avoid extremes. Thinness is a major risk factor for hip fractures associated with osteoporosis, while obesity increases the risk of or exacerbates disorders such as diabetes, heart disease, and hypertension.

CAN YOU BE TOO THIN?

Many people aspire to be thin, but contrary to the image increasingly portrayed by fashion and the media, thinness does not always mean you are fit and healthy. Being underweight can also place physical and psychological strains on the body.

Health risks of being underweight

As someone loses weight, symptoms such as fatigue and lethargy may appear. These are part of the body's natural response to starvation; it conserves energy by decreasing the energy output involved in all voluntary physical activity.

In children, being underweight can stunt growth and delay puberty—problems that can be irreversible. It is therefore vital that children are given a healthy, balanced diet and discouraged from any form of dieting, except under the advice and care of a doctor.

In women, being underweight can cause menstrual and fertility problems; below a certain weight women do not menstruate at all and are infertile. Older women who are too thin tend to suffer more from osteoporosis, and there may be some justification for doctors recommending postmenopausal women to be slightly plump rather than too thin. The risk of ill health increases below a BMI of 19 (see page 25). A BMI of less than 12 is generally fatal. If you are seriously underweight, for example, your BMI is less than 16, or if you are losing weight without trying and the reason is hard to pinpoint, consult your doctor, as it may be a sign of an underlying disease.

Causes of being underweight

There are a number of reasons for being underweight; some are straightforward, others are more complex.

A disorder of the thyroid gland, which helps to regulate the body's energy levels, can lead to the overproduction of thyroid hormones. This condition, called hyperthy-roidism (see page 34), can produce a range of symptoms, including weight loss. Food allergies and intolerances can also cause weight loss. Many food intolerances produce symptoms such as indigestion and nausea, which reduce appetite. An intolerance to gluten can lead to celiac disease, characterized by diarrhea and weight loss.

Any physical illness that includes trauma, inflammation, infection, or repair to tissues can lead to weight loss, mainly because of a decrease in appetite. With appropriate care, weight loss can be prevented or at least minimized. Sometimes it is possible to identify a specific cause, such as drugs that induce nausea or vomiting, but often the reason is difficult to pinpoint. If you suffer from more than a temporary loss of appetite, consult your primary-care doctor or a dietitian.

Stress and depression can also result in appetite loss and digestive problems such as nausea and irritable bowel syndrome. Depression, which often signals deeper emotional problems, may lead in extreme cases to the eating disorders anorexia nervosa or bulimia (see page 39). Anorexia nervosa, characterized by severe weight loss, can be fatal. People who are bulimic tend not to show such extreme weight loss as sufferers of anorexia, but they may still be underweight. Their repeated bouts of self-induced vomiting can lead to other health problems as well (see page 42).

Gaining weight

The best way to gain weight is to increase the size and number of meals you consume and their nutrient density. If you have been underweight for a significant period, however, your body may find it difficult to cope with large amounts of food at any one time. It is usually advisable to start by increasing the frequency of meals gradually, day by day, over a few weeks.

Your weight gain plan needs to be well thought out. It is important to keep the balance of food right and not be tempted by high-fat, calorie-laden foods in the hope of putting on weight quickly. You can eat healthfully and still increase your calorie intake. Make sure you have a good mixture of whole-grain cereals, fruit, and vegetables, and moderate amounts of meat and dairy foods (see pages 51–52) to maintain the right balance of vitamins, minerals, protein, and fiber necessary for good health.

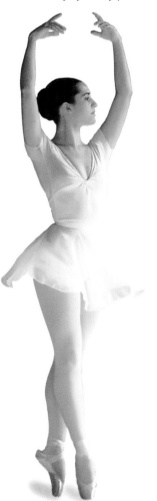

MUSCLE POWER
Ballet dancers are typically very thin, so how do they stay healthy at such a low weight? The answer is that a large proportion of their body weight is highly toned muscle, and they work out intensively almost every day to remain physically fit.

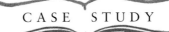

The Diabetes Sufferer

Diabetes that develops in adult life is known as non-insulin-dependent, because it can usually be treated without injections of insulin. Although insulin production is normal, the tissues of the body become unresponsive to it, and the typical symptoms of diabetes ensue. Being overweight compounds the problem, as high levels of fatty tissue further reduce the effect of insulin.

Mary is a 64-year-old, retired factory worker with a fairly sedentary lifestyle and a weight problem. She usually skips breakfast and snacks all day, preferring fried foods and meat to grilled or steamed foods and vegetables. Recently she has noticed that she tires more easily, particularly in the morning, and has found herself going to the toilet more often while also feeling very thirsty all the time. She became really worried when she had a dizzy spell, followed by blurred vision and a feeling of numbness in her hands and legs. She went to see her doctor, who diagnosed her as having adult-onset, or non-insulin-dependent, diabetes. He not only prescribed her a course of drug treatment but also referred her to a nutritionist.

WHAT SHOULD MARY DO?

Non-insulin-dependent diabetes can often be controlled through diet and exercise. To achieve this, Mary must first replace the sugar in her diet with a steady supply of complex carbohydrates, which will balance the glucose levels in her blood. She also needs to consume more soluble fiber to regulate her body's absorption of carbohydrates. The nutritionist recommends that she never skip a meal, include more legumes, vegetables, and whole grains in her meals as the basis for a high fiber, low-fat diet, and rely less on animal foods for protein. This program will also help her lose some weight, especially if she incorporates regular exercise into her daily life.

Action Plan

DIET
Eat beans, fruits, vegetables, and whole-grain cereals for carbohydrates and fiber. Take brewer's yeast for chromium, which helps the body metabolize glucose.

HEALTH
Seek medical advice. Treatment may be with drugs, followed by a consultation with a nutritionist to introduce new eating habits. Start an exercise program.

EATING HABITS
Eat regular, evenly spaced meals and replace sugary snacks with complex carbohydrates. Monitor blood glucose levels regularly.

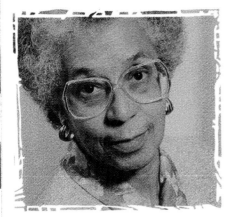

EATING HABITS
Skipping meals can lower blood sugar to dangerous levels.

DIET
Missing out on complex carbohydrates, fiber, and vital minerals like chromium can worsen diabetic symptoms.

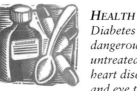

HEALTH
Diabetes can be very dangerous if left untreated, leading to heart disease, kidney and eye problems, and neurological disorders.

HOW THINGS TURNED OUT FOR MARY

Mary did change her diet and by eating regular, healthful meals, has weaned herself off drugs but still remains under medical supervision. She has also begun swimming twice a week and regularly takes long walks. Exercise has improved her circulation and mitigated the numbness in her hands and legs. Diet and exercise have also helped her lose several pounds. Instead of feeling tired she now has more energy than before.

Do you need to lose weight?

Losing weight can be beneficial to both health and mental well-being. Before starting a weight-loss plan, however, it's essential to assess the need for it objectively and to set realistic goals.

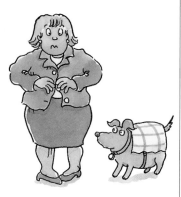

IT'S A TIGHT FIT!
Tight clothing is often the first sign of a need to lose weight. Many people face the dilemma of deciding whether to buy a new wardrobe or shed a few pounds.

Although losing weight is not easy, it can be a worthwhile endeavor if it improves appearance and boosts self-esteem. Of even greater benefit to anyone who strives to achieve an ideal weight, however, are decreased risks for the diseases associated with being overweight and increased levels of energy.

DETERMINING IF IT IS NECESSARY TO LOSE WEIGHT

For some people, deciding to diet can be simply a matter of finding that favorite clothes no longer fit. This may indeed be a valid indication of the need to eat less food. However, an increase in activity might be all that is needed; for example, exercises that tone the stomach muscles may help if waistbands have grown a little too tight.

If you do toning exercises regularly and still look fat, you probably are overweight. To determine if you have too much body fat, a doctor may use calipers, instruments that measure the thickness of a skinfold—the amount of skin and underlying fatty tissue that can be pinched together. About 50 percent of body fat lies just below the skin; thus skinfolds more than an inch thick on the underarm or area just above your hip bone usually indicate excess body fat. An even more accurate measurement of body fat is obtained by underwater weighing. You are weighed on land and again while submerged in water. A formula based on these two weights gives the percentage of body fat.

The Body Mass Index is another good way to determine if weight is healthy. The chart on page 25 shows you how to calculate it. If you are obese—if your BMI is over 30 (see page 25)—your health will benefit from even modest but sustained weight loss. If you have a BMI between 25 and 30, weight loss is advisable when other health risk factors are present, for example, if you are a heavy smoker or drinker or suffer from hypertension or diabetes.

Health risks of being obese

The main cause of premature death among obese people is heart disease: hypertension, coronary thrombosis, and congestive heart failure are all significantly more common among obese people than among those of healthy weight. In fact, obesity in women is one of the best predictors of cardiovascular disease, because excessive weight increases some important risk factors for it. Specifically, being overweight raises levels of cholesterol and triglycerides and increases blood pressure.

BURNING OFF CALORIES: *Swimming*

Swimming is an excellent cardio-respiratory exercise. It tones many areas of the body and, since it is non-weight-bearing, is ideal for pregnant women and people who have joint or back pain.

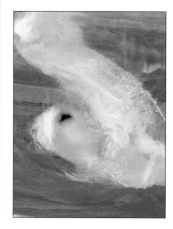

MUSCLE GROUPS BENEFITING
Helps strengthen the back and abdominal muscles. Works the upper arms and pectoral muscles. Breast stroke also works the thighs.

EQUIPMENT
Goggles will prevent eye irritation from chlorine or salt water.

CALORIES BURNED
Twenty minutes of continuous swimming will burn about 170 calories.

Non-insulin-dependent diabetes mellitus, or NIDDM, is also a major cause of death in obese people. A man who is more than 40 percent above his average weight is 5.2 times more likely to die of diabetes than a man of healthy weight; for women the ratio is 7.9 for a similar degree of excess weight.

Obese people are also more likely to develop gallstones, because their bile and excess adipose tissue (the body's connective tissue that stores fat) contain a lot of cholesterol.

Adipose tissue is a source of aromatase, the enzyme system that converts androgens (male sex hormones) to estrogens (female sex hormones). Consequently, obese people have a higher circulating level of estrogens compared with people of healthy weight. This possibly explains why obese women have more menstrual problems, a higher incidence of infertility, and irregular periods. It may also explain the increased prevalence of sex-hormone-sensitive cancers in obese women, such as malignant tumors of the breast, ovary, endometrium, and cervix.

Psychological consequences

People who are overweight often suffer more from depression and low self-esteem than those of healthy weight. The strength of the stigma and distress associated with being overweight was illustrated by a study conducted in the United States in 1991. It looked at the morbid fear of weight regain in patients who had once been obese but after special surgery had lost weight and successfully maintained this weight loss for at least three years. In spite of the strong tendency for people to evaluate their own worst handicap as less disabling than other handicaps, patients said they would prefer to be an ideal weight with a major handicap —being deaf, dyslexic, diabetic, legally blind, or having very bad acne, heart disease, or even one leg amputated—than to be extremely obese. All patients said they would rather be an ideal weight with the income they have now than an extremely obese multimillionaire.

Feelings of embarrassment and self-hate about being overweight can lead to reduced physical activity and an increased feeling of isolation and insularity, which may cause a slide into depression.

Severely obese people can have difficulties in social situations, too, because of their physical size. If they cannot fit into normal size chairs, they are virtually excluded from attending the theater or cinema or even traveling by public transportation unless they stand. These penalties all lead to an increase in the social isolation already felt by obese persons.

PHYSICAL RISKS OF BEING OVERWEIGHT

In addition to increasing risks for disease, being very overweight can also have harmful physical effects on your body.

▶ *Undue pressure placed on weight-bearing joints like hips and knees can result in osteoarthritis.*

▶ *Extra strain is placed on the heart, indicated by shortness of breath and general lethargy.*

▶ *Too much strain is placed on the back. Backaches are common, and existing back problems are exacerbated.*

▶ *There is an increase in the risks associated with anesthesia and surgery.*

WILL LOSING WEIGHT BENEFIT YOUR HEALTH?

Before you begin a weight-loss program, consider the reasons behind your decision. An important rationale for choosing to lose weight is to benefit your health and well-being. If you are overweight, factors such as smoking and too little exercise add to your health risks and make it even more beneficial to consider going on a diet. This quiz can help you determine if weight loss is appropriate for you. Score 4 each time you answer (a), 2 each time you answer (b), and 1 each time you answer (c). If none of the answers applies, score 0. Whatever your score, improving your diet and increasing your exercise can't help but improve your fitness.

QUESTIONS	ANSWERS		
IS YOUR BMI (SEE PAGE 25):	(a) 30 or over	(b) Between 25 and 30	(c) Below 25
DO YOU HAVE ANY OF THE FOLLOWING MEDICAL PROBLEMS:	(a) High cholesterol, high blood pressure, or diabetes	(b) Shortage of breath	(c) Indigestion or heartburn
DO YOU SMOKE CIGARETTES:	(a) Heavily – 20 or more a day	(b) Socially – 10 a day	(c) Seldom
IS YOUR WAIST-TO-HIP RATIO (SEE PAGE 24):	(a) 1.0 or above (man); 0.85 or above (woman)	(b) 0.95 or above (man); 0.75 or above (woman)	(c) Below 0.95 (man); below 0.75 (woman)
DO YOU EXERCISE FOR 20 MINUTES OR MORE:	(a) Seldom or never	(b) Once or twice a week	(c) More than twice a week
HOW DID YOU SCORE?	12–20: weight loss is advisable for health reasons.	8–12: weight loss may improve your general health.	Below 8: you probably do not need to lose weight.

Waist-to-hip ratio

Waist-to-hip ratio is a useful guide to whether the distribution of fat in your body is healthy. A waist-to-hip ratio above 1.0 in men; and above 0.85 in women is a sign of unhealthy fat distribution, which can increase the risk of many disorders, including heart disease.

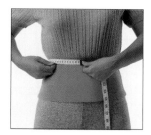

1 Measure your waist —the point just above the top of your hip bones where your body naturally curves inward.

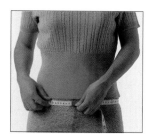

2 Measure your hips at their widest point— usually 7 to 9 inches below the waist. To calculate your waist-to-hip ratio, divide your waist measurement by your hip measurement.

DECIDING TO LOSE WEIGHT

Health is a very good reason for losing weight; if a health problem is sufficiently serious, many people find the motivation to reach a sensible weight and stay there. A particular health concern is carrying more fat around your stomach and waist than on your thighs and buttocks (see left for how to measure this ratio). Statistics show that this distribution increases the possibilities of heart disease, high blood pressure, arthritis, and non-insulin-dependent diabetes.

Losing weight in order to feel more attractive is also a good motivator but a more complicated issue. There may be a deeper emotional or psychological problem behind the desire to lose weight that needs looking at before a weight-control program can be successful. A recent study revealed that obesity is sometimes a "coat rack" where patients hang all their problems, failings, and unhappy feelings. Some obese patients who have lost weight subsequently found that the results and rewards they anticipated did not materialize, and life's problems continued and even intensified. Because challenges and difficulties in life are too complex to be resolved simply by a change in image, a weight-loss program may be doomed to failure when the goal is too high to be realistically achieved.

Some people wrongly assume that they are a healthy weight when they aren't. Correct assessment is essential (see page 22). Studies have shown that most men believe they are taller and more muscular than they really are, and most women think they are slimmer than is actually the case.

You will notice that there is no allowance for frame size in the BMI chart on page 25. It is a myth that big bones make a person significantly heavier—muscles, however, do. People who are particularly muscular can be healthy at higher weights than persons of average body composition; it is excess fat that is a problem.

HOW DO YOU LOSE WEIGHT?

The key to weight loss is shifting the balance so that energy (calorie) intake is less than energy expenditure. When this happens, weight loss will occur without fail. The way most people achieve this is to consume fewer calories and exercise more.

Even exercise alone will help you lose weight. For example, your body will start to burn fat after you have been performing any kind of aerobic activity for at least 20 minutes, and will continue to burn calories at a higher rate for several hours after you stop exercising. Exercise will also increase the proportion of lean tissue to fat in your body and, in turn, increase your metabolic rate.

Many people have reported that regular sustained exercise suppresses their appetite, both during and immediately afterward. Exactly why this happens is not fully understood, but one theory is that instense activity may normalize levels of insulin and other hormones that can influence appetite. Even if you don't experience this effect, you still benefit, because even small amounts of exercise assist in burning energy. Therefore, your diet doesn't need to be severe for you to start losing weight. Dieting will, in fact, lower your metabolic rate, and exercise will help balance this effect. Exercise will also improve your health in general and enhance your muscle tone and appearance.

Dieting without undertaking exercise may lead to only short-term weight loss. Exercise has been shown to be particularly important in maintaining a steady weight once the initial excess has been lost. As stated above, you can have a more normal diet without drastic eating restrictions, because regular exercise burns off more calories.

WEIGHT MEASUREMENT

Always weigh yourself first thing in the morning, right after going to the toilet. Use the same scale throughout your weight-control program, as scales can vary widely, even those in doctors' offices and hospitals.

GETTING IT RIGHT Make sure your scale is accurate and placed on a hard, level surface.

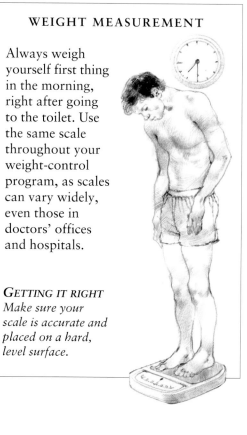

THE BODY MASS INDEX

Calculate your Body Mass Index from this table by locating your weight at the side and lining it up with your height. (See page 17 for converting kilograms and centimeters to pounds and inches.) A BMI greater than 25 is defined as being overweight. If your BMI is over 30, your health could be at risk; see your doctor.

WEIGHT (kg)	HEIGHT (cm)																
	150	152.5	155	157.5	160	162.5	165	167.5	170	172.5	175	177.5	180	182.5	185	187.5	190
40	18	17	17	16	16	15	15	14	14	13	13	13	12	12	12	11	11
41	18	18	17	17	16	16	15	15	14	14	13	13	13	12	12	12	11
42	19	18	17	17	16	16	15	15	15	14	14	13	13	13	12	12	12
43	19	18	18	17	17	16	16	15	15	14	14	14	13	13	13	12	12
44	20	19	18	18	17	17	16	16	15	15	14	14	14	13	13	13	12
45	20	19	19	18	18	17	17	16	16	15	15	14	14	14	13	13	12
46	20	20	19	19	18	17	17	16	16	15	15	15	14	14	13	13	13
47	21	20	20	19	18	18	17	17	16	16	15	15	15	14	14	13	13
48	21	21	20	19	19	18	18	17	17	16	16	15	15	14	14	14	13
49	22	21	20	20	19	19	18	17	17	16	16	16	15	15	14	14	14
50	22	21	21	20	20	19	18	18	17	17	16	16	15	15	15	14	14
51	23	22	21	21	20	19	19	18	18	17	17	16	16	15	15	15	14
52	23	22	21	20	20	20	19	19	18	17	17	17	16	16	15	15	14
53	24	23	22	21	21	20	19	19	18	18	17	17	16	16	15	15	15
54	24	23	22	22	21	20	20	19	19	18	18	17	17	16	16	15	15
55	24	24	23	22	21	21	20	20	19	18	18	17	17	17	16	16	15
56	25	24	23	23	22	21	21	20	19	19	18	18	17	17	16	16	16
57	25	25	24	23	22	22	21	20	20	19	19	18	18	17	17	16	16
58	26	25	24	23	23	22	21	21	20	19	19	18	18	17	17	16	16
59	26	25	25	24	23	22	22	21	20	20	19	19	18	18	17	17	16
60	27	26	25	24	23	23	22	21	21	20	20	19	19	18	18	17	17
61	27	26	25	25	24	23	22	22	21	20	20	19	19	18	18	17	17
62	28	27	26	25	24	23	23	22	21	21	20	20	19	19	18	18	17
63	28	27	26	25	25	24	23	22	22	21	21	20	19	19	18	18	17
64	28	28	27	26	25	24	24	23	22	22	21	20	20	19	19	18	18
65	29	28	27	26	25	25	24	23	22	22	21	21	20	20	19	18	18
66	29	28	27	27	26	25	24	24	23	22	22	21	20	20	19	19	18
67	30	29	28	27	26	25	25	24	23	23	22	21	21	20	20	19	19
68	30	29	28	27	27	26	25	24	24	23	22	22	21	20	20	19	19
69	31	30	29	28	27	26	25	25	24	23	23	22	21	21	20	20	19
70	31	30	29	28	27	27	26	25	24	24	23	22	22	21	20	20	19
71	32	31	30	29	28	27	26	25	25	24	23	23	22	21	21	20	20
72	32	31	30	29	28	27	26	26	25	24	24	23	22	21	21	20	20
73	32	31	30	29	29	28	27	26	25	25	24	23	23	22	21	21	20
74	33	32	31	30	29	28	27	26	26	25	24	23	23	22	22	21	20
75	33	32	31	30	29	28	28	27	26	25	24	24	23	23	22	21	21
76	34	33	32	31	30	29	28	27	26	26	25	24	23	23	22	22	21
77	34	33	32	31	30	29	28	27	27	26	25	24	24	23	22	22	21
78	35	34	32	31	30	30	29	28	27	26	25	25	24	23	23	22	22
79	35	34	33	32	31	30	29	28	27	27	26	25	24	24	23	22	22
80	36	34	33	32	31	30	29	29	28	27	26	26	25	24	24	23	22
81	36	35	34	33	32	31	30	29	28	27	26	26	25	24	24	23	22
82	36	35	34	33	32	31	30	29	28	28	27	26	25	25	24	23	23
83	37	36	35	33	32	31	30	30	29	28	27	26	26	25	24	24	23
84	37	36	35	34	33	32	31	30	29	28	27	27	26	25	25	24	23
85	38	37	35	34	33	34	31	30	29	29	28	27	26	26	25	24	24
86	38	37	36	35	34	33	32	31	30	30	28	28	27	26	25	24	24
87	39	37	36	35	34	33	32	31	30	29	28	28	27	26	25	25	24
88	39	38	37	35	34	33	32	31	30	30	29	28	27	26	26	25	24
89	40	38	37	36	35	34	33	32	31	30	29	28	27	27	26	25	25
90	40	39	37	36	35	34	33	32	31	30	29	29	28	27	26	26	25
91	40	39	38	37	36	34	33	32	31	31	30	29	28	27	27	26	25
92	41	40	38	37	36	35	34	33	32	31	30	29	28	28	27	26	25
93	41	40	39	37	36	35	34	33	32	31	30	30	29	28	27	26	26
94	42	40	39	38	37	36	35	34	33	32	31	30	29	28	27	27	26
95	42	41	40	38	37	36	35	34	33	32	31	30	29	29	28	27	26
96	43	41	40	39	38	36	35	34	33	32	31	30	30	29	28	27	27
97	43	42	40	39	38	37	36	35	34	33	32	31	30	29	28	28	27
98	44	42	41	40	38	37	36	35	34	33	32	31	30	29	29	28	27
99	44	43	41	40	39	37	36	35	34	33	32	31	31	30	29	28	27
100	44	43	42	40	39	38	37	36	35	34	33	32	31	30	29	28	28

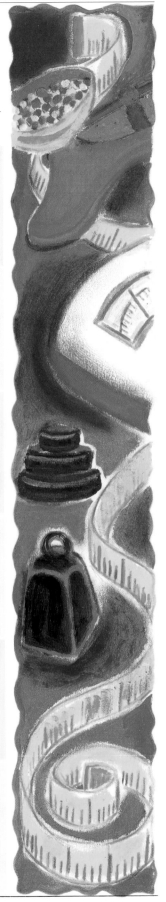

How much weight should you expect to lose each week?

Losing weight is a slow process. If you consume 1000 calories per day less than you expend, then you should lose 0.5 kg to 1 kg (1 to 2 lb) per week. This represents a healthy and sustainable weight loss. Don't be discouraged if your weight loss is no greater than this. Many people give up on a diet because in their view it is not working, but losing a large amount of weight fast can have health risks, is harder to sustain, and is likely to be regained.

What is a calorie?

The unit of measure used to describe the energy content of foods is called a calorie. However, as a calorie is so small, it has become normal to talk in measures of 1,000, or kilocalories. Health and nutrition experts sometimes use Calorie (with a capital C) and abbreviate to kcal or cal. In common usage, kilocalorie is shortened to calorie or cal.

Therapies and surgical intervention

For some seriously obese people, a more drastic approach is sometimes prescribed for weight loss. There are many drugs for the treatment of obesity, but these do have potential side effects, including nervousness, high blood pressure, palpitations, dizziness, headaches, insomnia, mood swings, tremor, dry mouth, diarrhea, constipation, itching, and rashes. In the short term, appetite suppressants (or anorectic drugs) help with weight loss, but patients often regain the weight when they stop taking the drugs. Also, these medications have a potential for addiction. Some patients may be given drugs that not only suppress appetite but also speed up their metabolic rate. Unfortunately, all such drugs gradually lose their effectiveness because the body builds up a tolerance for them.

Surgical procedures include gastric stapling and gastric bypass. In gastric stapling a line of staples is punched through the stomach so that only about 50 ml (1¾ fl oz) of food can be taken at any one time. A gastric bypass is an operation in which the gut is cut and rejoined to provide a relatively short exposure of food to the action of digestive enzymes, while the majority of the bowel is short-circuited. This means that less food is actually absorbed by the body. Weight loss is usually rapid following these operations, but they are not without risks; metabolic disorders and other serious health problems can result. Such drastic measures are recommended only for severely obese people for whom other weight-loss measures have failed, and ongoing medical supervision is necessary.

One of the more successful treatments for weight control is behavioral therapy. The idea behind this approach is that eating habits are learned and that obese people have learned a type of eating behavior that leads to weight gain. Behavioral therapy helps a person change to new eating patterns. For example, for a patient who binge eats, the key to success is to identify what triggers these binges and work from there, either by avoiding the triggers or learning how to deal with them in a way that doesn't involve eating. As with all weight management programs, behavioral therapy is most successful when it is combined with lifelong changes to eating habits and a permanent increase in physical activity.

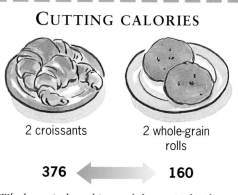

CUTTING CALORIES

2 croissants	2 whole-grain rolls
376	160

Whole-grain bread is much lower in fat than a croissant and is a better source of fiber.

Diet and weight control for everyone

For anyone embarking on a diet and exercise program, the aim should be weight control rather than dramatic weight loss in the short term. Set yourself a realistic target weight but also set a number of interim targets. The goal is often so far away from the starting point that without small victories along the way, you may be tempted to give up as you realize the long and difficult task before you. It is much better to lose a little weight slowly and keep it off, than to lose a significant amount quickly only to regain it.

People who are constantly on diets (yo-yo dieters) and whose weight fluctuates over time are at greater risk for ill health. They often experience a significantly lower sense of general well-being and greater stress than those who maintain a healthy weight. Furthermore, there is some evidence that yo-yo dieting may make an overweight patient more vulnerable to binge behavior. Maintaining a stable weight after weight loss should be seen as just as important as the initial loss of weight.

The key to successful long-term weight maintenance is to make small but significant and permanent changes to your diet and activity level. Keep a food diary so that you can assess if your diet delivers all of the nutrients your body needs and in the correct proportions (see page 51). Look at ways to reduce fat, such as substituting low-fat alternatives for high-fat dairy products and grilling, broiling, or steaming food instead of frying it. Improve your fitness level by gradually increasing the amount of aerobic exercise you do (see Chapter 5) until you are exercising for at least 20 minutes or more, 3 to 5 times a week.

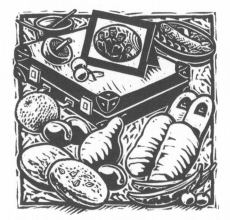

CHAPTER 2

WHY IS YOUR BODY THE SHAPE IT IS?

Weight is influenced by several factors that interact in complex ways. The primary controlling factor is the energy content of the food we eat in relation to our energy requirements, but other functions such as metabolism, genetics, feelings, and the environment all play important roles.

THE PHYSIOLOGY OF WEIGHT CONTROL

Weight is affected by the interaction of a number of physiological factors—including appetite, metabolism, hormones, and heredity—most of which can be influenced by your actions.

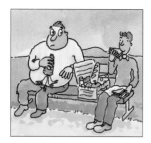

CAUSE AND EFFECT
Regular exercise expends more energy than a sedentary lifestyle and burns off extra calories instead of storing them as fat. This means the calorie intake of an active person can be higher than that of someone who is inactive.

Many physiological functions have contributed to making you the weight you are now. Some, such as your genetic make-up, you have no control over. But there are other areas, for example, your body's metabolism, in which you can implement change for the better.

HUNGER AND APPETITE

It is important to understand the difference between hunger and appetite in order to control the factors that make you want to eat. Hunger is a physiological message sent by your body to alert you to the fact that food is required for your survival. It occurs when the stomach is empty and blood sugar levels are running low. Appetite, on the other hand, is a desire for and an anticipation of food that may not reflect a physical need for it. Even before food enters the mouth, the sight and smell causes the stomach and intestines to prepare for it. Appetite can override the fact that hunger has been satisfied and so has an important role in the amount of energy taken into the body through food and drink. Endorphins, the body's natural painkillers and mood elevators, may also play a part in appetite. Studies show that higher levels of endorphins are released in obese people after they have eaten. This may explain why such persons appear to be addicted to food.

How the body senses satiety

The body's regulatory mechanisms are self-programmed to ensure that it gets enough fuel (calories) by initiating the drive to eat whenever it has an under supply of energy.

HOW THE BRAIN CONTROLS APPETITE

Appetite is regulated by a part of the brain called the hypothalamus, which monitors appetite factors such as the levels of glucose (sugar) and other chemicals in the blood. It also receives signals from stretch sensors in the stomach, which indicate if it is empty or full. The hypothalamus thus stimulates the drive to eat when necessary. Following a meal these appetite factors subside and the hypothalamus sends out satiety signals, which suppress the appetite. These signals are slower to work, however, which can lead to overeating.

Hypothalamus monitors the status of appetite factors and gut stretch sensors and activates or suppresses appetite.

Salivary glands release saliva containing digestive enzymes, to begin food breakdown.

Liver stores excess sugar following a meal and slowly releases it as needed by the body.

BRAIN CONTROL
Appetite involves a complex system that is regulated by a tiny region of the brain.

Olfactory (smell) nerves and taste buds detect the presence of food and activate salivary glands and digestive enzymes in the stomach.

Stomach releases digestive enzymes to continue food breakdown. Stretch receptors indicate when the stomach is full.

Small intestine detects food leaving stomach and produces digestive enzymes to continue food breakdown. Absorbs nutrients into bloodstream.

But the opposing mechanism to stop eating when enough energy has been consumed, does not appear to operate quite so effectively; overeating does not produce powerful signals to cut down. Numerous studies have demonstrated that if we have access to an abundant supply of palatable, high-fat food we tend to overeat. This is known as "passive over-consumption," which means that we continue to eat the same amount of food, but the calorie intake is much higher because fat is more energy dense than carbohydrate or protein.

The body's weak defences against overeating means that most people find it easy to do. Undereating, however, requires more effort and willpower and is usually a deliberate act, unless a person is ill.

METABOLISM

The process by which food is broken down to release energy is known as metabolism. The energy is used to perform various functions, such as keeping the heart beating, maintaining liver function, and providing fuel for exercise and other physical activity.

If your weight is stable, then the amount of fuel (measured in calories or joules) you are taking in is equal to the amount you are using for energy. If you eat too much, the extra is stored as fat. To lose weight you must eat fewer calories than you burn off.

How much energy your body uses depends on a number of factors. The main determinant is the Basal Metabolic Rate (BMR). This is the amount of energy used by the body for functions such as breathing, making the heart beat, and producing heat. In other words it is the amount needed to keep you living. This fuel factor is influenced by age, gender, body size, and nutritional and physical status as well as genetics. You also use up additional energy during physical activity and exercise.

What affects metabolism

The amount of exercise you do is the main influence on the body's metabolic rate. The more active you are, the faster your metabolism will be and the more energy you will burn. In time, with regular exercise, it is possible to increase your resting metabolic rate so that your body uses more energy for every action from breathing to sports.

A number of substances can also induce a change in the amount of energy the body uses. Nicotine and caffeine cause small but measurable increases in the metabolic rate. Agents such as amphetamines, thyroxine, and some drugs used in the treatment of obesity cause an increase. too.

Other drugs reduce energy expenditure. Among them are beta-blockers and drugs used in the treatment of angina and hypertension, for the prevention of migraine, and to control an overactive thyroid gland. These may even produce a slight weight gain.

Certain illnesses can increase the body's metabolic rate. For example, in Graves disease the thyroid gland is overactive, making the body use more energy than normal. The metabolic rate increases in response to stress and fear as well.

Raising your metabolism

Exercise will increase your metabolic rate, but to make significant changes that alter your body composition you need to exercise on a regular basis—not for one post-holiday session that puts a sudden strain on the heart and leads to aching muscles. Moderate exercise for 20 to 30 minutes every other day is more beneficial than an intensive one-hour workout once a week.

It is important to fit exercise into your daily life and find forms that you enjoy, so it doesn't become a boring task. Besides planned workouts, there are simple ways to introduce more activity. Ask yourself do you really need to ride a bus for only three stops? Must you take the elevator up two floors? Could you go out for a walk at lunch time?

There are no foods that will burn off fat; it is a misconception that grapefruit, herbs, or other products will melt fat away or boost metabolism. Also without scientific foundation are claims that a special mixture of foods when taken in a certain way will have a magical effect, or that a particular mix of nutrients will increase your energy output. Such diets work only if they help you restrict total calorie intake.

Unfortunately, even dieting itself lowers your metabolic rate. When your intake of food drops, your metabolic rate slows down to enable you to function while using as little energy and stored fat as possible. This is the continued on page 32

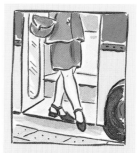

QUICK FITNESS TIP
Get off the bus two stops before you normally do and walk the rest of the way.

HIGH ENERGY NEEDS
After years of following strenuous training regimens, athletes develop such a high metabolic rate that they must consume large quantities of food every day just to keep pace with their energy needs.

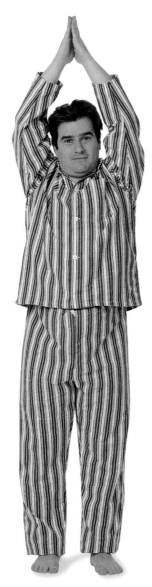

Exercising to boost your

Metabolism

There are positive steps you can take, from the moment you wake up in the morning until the end of the day, to boost your metabolism and raise your energy level. These activities are especially important if you spend a lot of time in a chair.

Regular exercise is needed to boost metabolism and keep it at a higher level. The exercises shown here are particularly suited to people who are sedentary most of the day. The movements can be practiced anywhere, anytime, without the need for a lot of space, expensive equipment, or much spare time. If you are sluggish or lethargic on waking or feel that you cannot function without constant caffeine boosts, these activities demonstrate that the best pick-me-up at any time is gentle exercise.

At first, you may find it difficult to stretch as far as you feel you should but don't worry; it is important not to push your muscles too far and to stop if you feel any pain. With daily perseverance you will quickly notice a marked improvement in your suppleness and energy levels, as well as in your mental agility.

It may be easier for you to adopt an exercise routine successfully if you get the support of your work colleagues. Encourage them to join in whenever possible.

7am As soon as you get out of bed, perform some simple stretches such as the two on this page to start your blood flowing and warm up joints and muscles. Try to hold each stretch for 8 to 10 seconds, but relax slowly if you begin to feel tense or sore.

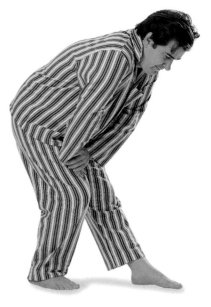

OVERHEAD STRETCH
Stand with your feet hip width apart, your back straight, and your head in line with your spine. Lift your arms above your head and reach as far upward as you can with your palms touching. To extend the stretch farther, ease your arms back slightly. Repeat five times.

HAMSTRING STRETCH
Stand with your feet apart. Keeping your chest lifted and your stomach pulled in, take a step forward with your left leg, keeping it straight. Bend your right knee and lean forward from the hips, lowering your chest toward your right thigh. Hold the stretch. Repeat with the other leg.

8am Find a more physically active way to get to work than driving your car, if possible. Can you walk to a railway station? If you catch a bus, can you walk briskly for 20 minutes to a bus stop farther from your home? Do some gentle

stretches as you walk—swing your arms and flex your fingers by alternately making fists and then opening them. You can also use this time to become aware of how your body feels as it moves and which movements work particular muscles.

9am At the office, use the stairs rather than the elevator to get to your floor and keep using the stairs throughout the day if you have to run errands between floors. Try to pace your climb so you are not exhausted at the end of it.

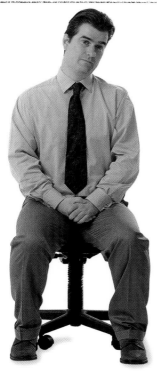

11 **am** Don't be tempted to have a doughnut or cake for your mid-morning break. Try this series of stretches instead. These movements are particularly important if you sit in front of a computer terminal most of the day, because muscles can become stiff if you remain in one position for long periods of time.

NECK STRETCH

Sitting with your back straight and your chest lifted, clasp your hands loosely in front of you and relax your shoulders. Keeping your shoulders still, slowly incline your left ear toward your left shoulder. When you have tilted your head as far as you can comfortably, hold the stretch. Repeat to the right side.

ARM STRETCH

Clasp your hands behind your back and slowly lift your arms up, keeping your elbows straight. Hold for a few seconds.

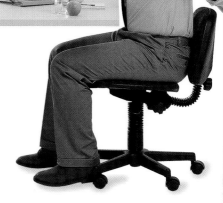

1 **pm** During the second half of your lunch hour, take time out for a brisk walk around the local streets. The change of scene will also serve to restore your concentration.

3 **pm** Mid-afternoon, perform more stretches, choosing ones that target different muscles from those worked on earlier. The two below are good for shoulders and triceps.

6 **pm** If your usual railway station or bus stop is close to your office, try walking to a station or stop a little farther away; or take a scenic route to the stop. You might even miss the worst of the rush hour crowds by taking a walk for 20 or 30 minutes after work, before you catch your bus or train home.

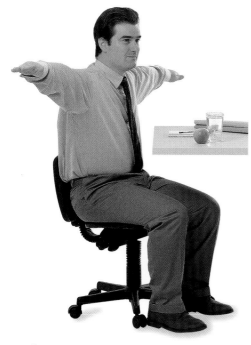

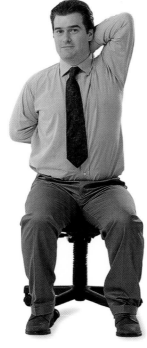

SHOULDER STRETCH

Keeping your arms level with your shoulders, extend them away from your body and reach out as far as is comfortable. Make small circles by rotating your arms backward five times and then forward five times.

TRICEP STRETCH

Place your left hand behind your back so that your palm sits between your shoulder blades and your elbow points upward. Bring your right hand up behind your back and try to join hands. Hold, then repeat with the other arm.

body's built-in protective mechanism against starvation. After being on a diet for two weeks, your metabolic rate can drop by as much as 10 percent. Exercise helps to prevent this fall, so it is crucial for successful weight loss. Dieting alone simply allows the body to become more efficient at functioning on less food.

Changes in metabolism over time

Metabolism can change during your lifetime due to a number of factors. There is a small decrease in BMR with age—1 to 2 percent up to the age of 60 and slightly more after that. But a much more significant contributor to a lower BMR is the gradual decrease in physical activity that usually occurs as people grow older. If you are not as active as you once were, then the amount of muscle in your body dwindles and you don't need as much energy. The weight gain associated with aging is often a result of the fact that diet has not changed even though energy expenditure has been reduced.

THE LIPOSTAT THEORY

There is a theory that the amount of fat in the body governs appetite and energy intake. The cornerstone to this theory is that the body has a preset genetically determined body fat mass. The sensors for this are in the brain, in particular, the hypothalamus, and in and around the appetite control centers. An unknown chemical released from the adipose tissue signals the hypothalamus about the state of the body's energy stores. To put it simply, it works like a central heating system. The hypothalamus is the thermostat for the sensors found in fat tissue. Depending on the state of the fat stores, it drives or suppresses appetite in an attempt to maintain their level. However, like any other thermostat it is not perfect, and small fluctuations in intake cannot be sensed. One theory is that even very few calories above your daily needs can lead to a large weight gain in the long term. This cannot be picked up by the thermostat initially, and the difference may be so slight that the thermostat resets itself. But when you want to lose weight and decrease your calorie intake substantially, the thermostat interprets the drop as a starvation warning and sends powerful signals that you are hungry.

HORMONES

Many hormones are involved in appetite control, and the number that have been identified grows constantly. Insulin is known to have an effect on appetite and weight, and thyroid hormones and sex hormones also play an important part.

The role of insulin

Two hormones produced by the pancreas control blood sugar levels in the body. Glucagon stimulates the breakdown of carbohydrates stored in the liver and muscles into glucose, or sugar, which is then released into the bloodstream. Insulin lowers blood sugar levels by stimulating the uptake of glucose by the body's cells. The theory that insulin and other hormones from the pancreas have a role in eating behavior is not new, but remains controversial.

Injection of a small amount of insulin produces a slight fall in blood glucose levels and this can trigger the urge to eat. The reason is probably that the hypothalamus detects the lower levels of glucose in the blood and initiates the desire to eat to make up the deficit. It is also possible that insulin plays a part in the satiety response. After eating, insulin levels drop in the brain as well as in the body tissues and this may play a part in inhibiting the desire to eat.

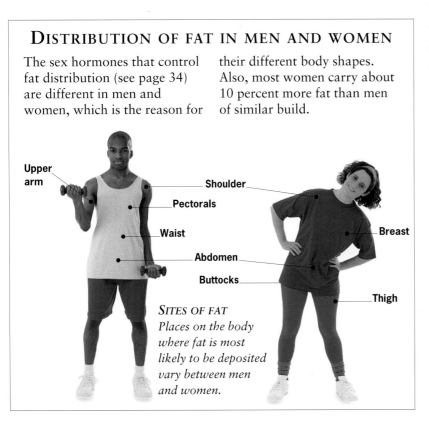

DISTRIBUTION OF FAT IN MEN AND WOMEN

The sex hormones that control fat distribution (see page 34) are different in men and women, which is the reason for their different body shapes. Also, most women carry about 10 percent more fat than men of similar build.

Upper arm

Shoulder

Pectorals

Waist

Breast

Abdomen

Buttocks

Thigh

SITES OF FAT
Places on the body where fat is most likely to be deposited vary between men and women.

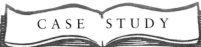
The Overweight Family

If all members of a family are overweight, this may indicate that there is a genetic predisposition to weight gain. But genetic make-up doesn't have to dictate weight. Changes in diet and exercise can enable individuals to overcome genetic influences and thus control their body shape and weight and effect major improvements in health and fitness.

Susan, 46, has recently returned to work after being a housewife and mother for 13 years. She has begun to feel self-conscious about her weight, because she has gained 19 kg (42 lb) over the past 10 years. Her husband has also mentioned that he feels uncomfortable about his weight. Susan knows that the children don't enjoy sports at school and realizes that they may be unhappy because of their weight, too. Susan has tried dieting before but has always put the weight back on. This time she has decided to make long-term changes in the lifestyle and eating habits of the whole family that will benefit them all. After talking to her doctor and doing some reading for ideas, Susan called a family conference.

WHAT SHOULD THE FAMILY DO?

Susan might begin by involving the whole family in meal planning. She herself needs to reduce the amount of fried foods that she prepares and use other cooking methods such as grilling and baking. Also, three to four nights a week she should substitute fish, poultry, or a vegetarian dish for their usual red meat. To control their habitual snacking in front of the television every evening, the family could try activities such as board games, which will distract them from the urge to snack. As family members don't do any physical exercise, this would be a good time to introduce joint activities like outdoor games, swimming, walks, or bicycle rides, which can be fun for both the adults and children.

Action Plan

EATING HABITS
Gradually decrease the amount of fat and sugar-laden foods from the family's meals and reduce evening snacking. Use fruit and vegetables as healthy snacks and substitute fruit for high-calorie desserts.

DIET
Roast, grill, or poach chicken and remove the skin. Bake potatoes in their jackets. Trim visible fat from meat and cut down on fried foods.

EXERCISE
Walk to and from school with the children to burn calories. Find an activity the whole family enjoys and make it a weekly event.

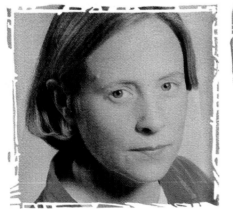

EATING HABITS
A diet that is high in fatty foods will not always satisfy hunger and can lead to the urge to reach for snacks, which often are also high in fat.

DIET
Untrimmed meat increases the fat content of a meal significantly. Cooking foods in fat adds extra calories.

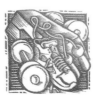

EXERCISE
Lack of exercise means little fat is burned as energy.

HOW THINGS TURNED OUT FOR THE FAMILY

Susan took time to plan meals around healthful eating principles. Also, instead of buying sweets, she made sure that there were always fruit, whole-grain crackers, and other healthy snack foods in the house. An evening cooking course gave her new recipe ideas. The family began swimming together regularly and, as they lost weight, the children started to show more interest in school sports. Over three months Susan lost 10 kg (22 lb) and her confidence at work increased.

CUTTING CALORIES

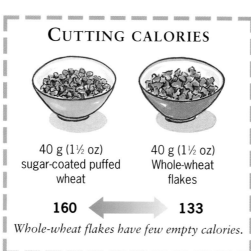

40 g (1½ oz)
sugar-coated puffed
wheat

40 g (1½ oz)
Whole-wheat
flakes

160 ⟷ **133**

Whole-wheat flakes have few empty calories.

Thyroid hormones

Thyroid hormones regulate the body's metabolism. Disorders that cause insufficient thyroid production, or hypothyroidism, can cause the body to put on weight, while overproduction of thyroid hormones, known as hyperthyroidism, can cause weight loss. Synthetic thyroid hormone drugs are used to treat both problems.

Although there have been some studies conducted on using thyroid hormones to help obese people lose weight, such treatments have generally not been successful because of the numerous side effects and excessive loss of lean tissue rather than fat.

Sex hormones

Male and female sex hormones control the distribution of fat. The male hormone testosterone concentrates fat around the stomach. Testosterone also appears to promote an increase in appetite in people who are taking it for therapeutic reasons. The female sex hormone estrogen concentrates fat distribution around the buttocks and thighs. Estrogen and fat are also strongly linked in that a certain amount of fat is necessary to enable the body to produce sufficient levels of estrogen. This is part of nature's way of ensuring that women have sufficient energy levels for reproduction.

Estrogen-containing pills such as oral contraceptives can lead to weight gain in some women, but why this occurs is not clear. Because the pill increases the level of estrogen in the body, it is thought that it further accentuates a woman's natural tendency to store excess fat. The hormone may also stimulate appetite.

Many women report weight gain after menopause. Again, exactly why this should happen is not clear. What is known is that a woman's fat distribution changes at this time due to a drop in estrogen levels, and that she is more likely to start putting on weight around the stomach rather than the buttocks and thighs (see page 19).

THE THYROID GLAND AND WEIGHT

An underactive or overactive thyroid gland can lead to some weight problems, however it is a misconception that these conditions are common. In fact, thyroid problems affect only about 1 percent of the adult population. Situated at the front of the neck, the thyroid is one of the main hormone glands that help regulate the body's energy levels. Correct production of thyroid hormones is crucial for promoting normal physical growth and mental development in children and for controlling metabolic rate.

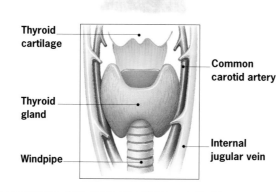

Thyroid cartilage

Thyroid gland

Windpipe

Common carotid artery

Internal jugular vein

HYPERTHYROIDISM
Overproduction of hormones by the thyroid gland causes symptoms such as fatigue, anxiety, sweating, intolerance to heat, diarrhea, palpitations, and weight loss. Treatment may involve partial removal of the gland, taking drugs to inhibit hormone production, or, especially in older people, a dose of radioactive iodine to destroy some of the thyroid tissue.

HYPOTHYROIDISM
An underactive thyroid gland leads to insufficient production of thyroid hormone, causing symptoms such as tiredness, dry skin, hair loss, sensitivity to cold, constipation, and weight gain. Treatment usually consists of prescribed doses of the thyroid hormone thyroxine, and this therapy generally has to be continued for the rest of the patient's life.

HEREDITY

There is little doubt that heredity has a role to play in determining weight, but just how large a part is still being debated. Considerable evidence exists for a genetic predisposition to obesity. Identical twins are twice as likely to have a similar height-to-weight ratio, or Body Mass Index (BMI), than are nonidentical twins. Studies show a relationship between the BMI of adult adoptees and their biological parents, but no correlation with their adoptive parents.

Genetic factors

Recently there has been much excitement about the discovery of a genetic fault in some mice that causes obesity. The mice with this fault do not produce enough of a protein called leptin, which appears to help control weight. A similar gene has been identified in humans, but the theory is complicated by the fact that obese people have more leptin in their blood than thin people do. This suggests that in humans the leptin being produced is not working effectively, whereas in obese mice insufficient leptin is the problem. This protein could be the previously unknown factor released from fat that has been identified in the Lipostat Theory (see page 32).

Although human trials of leptin have already begun, even if they are successful it will be many years before this knowledge leads to a new treatment for obesity. Moreover, there is probably no single gene that causes obesity in humans. Rather, a combination of genes is possibly involved, which makes identification much more difficult and makes it unlikely that any one treatment will help everyone.

Fetal nourishment

One of the discoveries made recently is that the nourishment a fetus receives may affect that person's health in later life. Professor David Barker and his team in Southampton, England, in the early 1990s studied birth records, including birth weight and length, of a group of people born in Herefordshire from 1911 onward. They were able to trace these people as adults and record their state of health, or discover their cause of death. The results showed that babies who were born at full term but weighed less than expected had more health problems later in life. One theory for this is that the mothers'

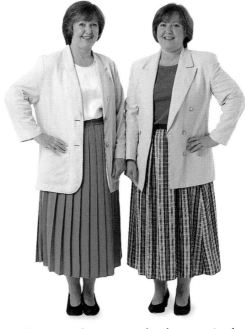

NATURE AND NURTURE
Identical twins are often the same weight and build when adults, even if raised by different parents. This shows the important part genes play in development.

poor diets may have caused a decrease in the number of cells formed in the pancreas, thus putting the infants at risk later for diabetes. The babies may also have adapted to their poor diets by becoming very efficient at storing nutrients, and later in life this may have led to a greater risk of diabetes and heart disease and, possibly, obesity.

Not all studies, however, show the same effect. There is probably an interplay between genetic susceptibility to disease, a baby's environment in the womb, and other events later in life that together determine the likelihood of chronic illnesses.

BURNING OFF CALORIES: *Cycling*

Cycling is a good all-around aerobic activity that can be used to develop cardiovascular fitness. As a low-impact exercise it can be especially beneficial to people with joint problems.

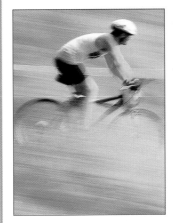

MUSCLE GROUPS BENEFITING
All of the leg muscles benefit, including the quadriceps (thigh muscle) and the gastrocnemius (calf muscle).

EQUIPMENT
A roadworthy bicycle and a bicycle helmet, or an indoor exercise bike.

CALORIES BURNT
At 16 km (10 miles) per hour, you expend 9 calories per minute: that's 540 calories per hour.

PSYCHOLOGICAL FACTORS

Your emotional state and the way you perceive yourself can have a direct influence on your weight; for many people it is often the determining factor in their weight problem.

Psychological factors play a major role in influencing your eating habits. Most people are aware that severe psychological disturbances are involved in the dieting disorders anorexia nervosa and bulimia; but milder emotional problems and perceptions can also affect everyday eating habits and weight in a variety of ways.

Research on eating disorders has revealed just how close the relationship is between one's psychological state and eating impulses. Anxiety, stress, and depression can lead both to appetite loss and to the opposite—

food cravings and binge eating. The foods most commonly craved are those that are sugar-laden and high in fat. Research indicates that these foods may increase mood-elevating chemicals in the brain.

Studies carried out between 1989 and 1991 by Dr. Ulrike Schmidt of the Institute of Psychiatry in London showed that there is a clear link between anxiety and stress and the development of anorexia and bulimia. Her studies also indicated that major life events such as a death in the family or a divorce precipitated the onset of eating disorders in

STEPS TOWARD A BETTER SELF-IMAGE

It is easy to become too focused on a desire to lose weight. You can quickly become overly critical of yourself and lose self-confidence or become depressed. If a weight-loss program is to be successful it must be fueled by conviction, and this requires a healthy self-image and the right motivation. Here are some suggestions on how to boost your self-esteem.

▶ *Read fashion magazines that portray glamorous models with a more critical eye. It is important to recognize that these images are highly stylized. Professional make-up, lighting, and camera angles are used to create the perfect images we see in periodicals and on television.*
▶ *Assess what is truly important in your life. Making a list of priorities in terms of career, travel, study, or relationship commitments can put body image into better perspective.*
▶ *Turn your attention toward something other than your weight. Weight loss is a long-term commitment; for a short-term confidence boost, try a new hair style or have a make-up lesson.*
▶ *Stop thinking negatively. If something negative comes to mind, write it down and then think of a positive statement to counteract it.*
▶ *Take time to look through your wardrobe and choose outfits that you feel good in. Opt for flattering styles that skim over problem areas like stomach and hips. Long-line jackets and blouses and long flowing skirts have a slimming effect.*

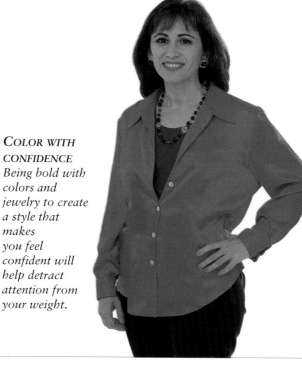

COLOR WITH CONFIDENCE *Being bold with colors and jewelry to create a style that makes you feel confident will help detract attention from your weight.*

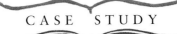

A Bulimia Sufferer

Between 2 and 4 percent of women are thought to have bulimia. Most of them keep it a secret. Although occasional overeating is perfectly normal, especially in a social setting, the loss of control over their eating habits that women with bulimia experience is not. It can be both distressing and harmful to their well-being, if kept up for a prolonged period of time.

Alice is 32 and lives on her own. She developed bulimia after divorcing her husband two years ago. Since her divorce she has suffered bouts of depression and has begun to feel increasingly lonely and isolated. Pressure at work has forced her to take on more tasks than she can cope with. As a result, she has been working very late and spending most evenings alone in her apartment. Although she used to be very active, since her work load increased she has not had time to go to the gym and has started missing meals to try to lose weight. The stress of work and her loneliness at home has led Alice to binge, and because of the resulting guilt and disgust she feels, she forces herself to vomit afterward.

WHAT SHOULD ALICE DO?

Alice needs to come to terms with the divorce from her husband and her other emotional needs. Consulting a counselor may help. She will have to recognize the link between her emotional health and her eating patterns.

She should also take steps to alleviate her sense of isolation at home. Setting aside time for doing things she enjoys, like going out with friends or seeing a film, is especially important whenever Alice feels like bingeing. Exercise may help boost her mood and relieve stress, so making time for gym sessions could also help. Learning to say no to extra tasks assigned by her supervisor is another important first step.

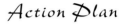

Action Plan

STRESS
Learn to relax: take a bath, listen to music, or become involved in an interesting pastime to alleviate stress.

EMOTIONAL HEALTH
Set up a meeting with a counselor to discuss and try to overcome detrimental emotions.

EATING HABITS
Eat three balanced meals a day and limit between-meal snacks to fruit, air-popped popcorn, and other low-fat foods to help control weight.

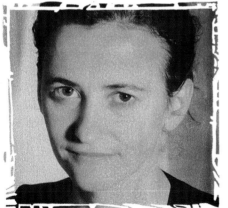

STRESS
Strain and stress often seem to play a role in bulimia. Developing effective ways of coping can reduce stress.

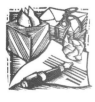

EMOTIONAL HEALTH
Emotional problems such as grief and depression are often associated with eating disorders.

EATING HABITS
Missing meals to lose weight makes people hungrier, which makes overeating more likely later on.

HOW THINGS TURNED OUT FOR ALICE

Alice negotiated a fairer distribution of the tasks at work and left earlier at night. She felt less tired, started enjoying her free time again, and began seeing a counselor, who made her feel more positive about herself after helping her see that the divorce was not all her fault. Her stress and boredom diminished and her health improved with regular meals. As she regained control of her eating, her bingeing and vomiting gradually stopped.

Yogic relaxation
Yogic techniques can reduce the stress that accompanies underlying problems related to food cravings and bingeing. Many community centers offer yoga classes. Once you have learned the basics, there are many techniques, such as deep abdominal breathing (see below), that you can practice at home.

MUDRA BREATHING
Sit on your calves with back straight. Link your hands behind your back and push your shoulders back. Breathe deeply. On every second exhalation slowly lower the torso from the hips, for as long as the exhalation lasts; keep your back straight. As you inhale, slowly rise. Repeat four times.

DO YOUR MOODS DICTATE YOUR EATING HABITS?

Breaking the link between your emotional state and your food intake can be the first step to successful weight control. Recognizing that there is an emotional dimension to your eating may help you adopt healthier eating habits. By learning the triggers to emotional eating, you can be prepared and either avoid these situations or have healthy snacks on hand. If you answer yes to one or more of the questions below, there may be an emotional factor affecting your eating habits.

QUESTIONS	YES	NO
Do you eat more when you are alone, for example, when watching television?		
Do you compensate yourself with cookies or other sweets if you've had a difficult day?		
If you've broken your diet and eaten a rich dessert, do you feel so upset that you might as well give up and eat what you like for the rest of the day?		
Does looking in the mirror or weighing yourself make you so depressed that you need a treat to cheer you up?		
Do you eat high-fat foods such as roasted nuts, potato chips, and chocolate to give yourself a boost when you're feeling down?		

75 percent of cases. A second study done by Nicholas Troop at the same institute from 1993 to 1995, found that women with eating disorders were less likely to respond well to stress and overcome the problems it posed than those without such disorders.

It is often difficult to establish exactly what has caused the anxious or depressed state. The loss of a loved one, work pressure, or relationship problems are obvious enough causes, but anxiety and depression can also result from more deep-seated psychological problems that may need to be examined with the help of a professional counselor.

Depression can in turn lead to nutritional deficiencies or imbalances, as sufferers often neglect their dietary needs or turn to high-fat or sugary foods for some sort of comfort. A lack of some micronutrients, particularly the B vitamins and C, can contribute to depression, and a vicious cycle of nutritional imbalance and depression may follow.

Dieting and depression
Early studies of women suffering from obesity suggested that the majority of sufferers overate in direct response to stress, anxiety, and depression. Later studies, however, have indicated that the relationship between appetite, eating habits, and emotional health is more complex than this. Research at the University of Toronto suggested that stress-induced overeating was actually a result of dieting. It was discovered that women who diet, and therefore restrain their desire for food, have two and a half times greater risk of developing eating disorders than nondieters. Dieters tend to have strict rules about eating. For example there are many foods that are described as "forbidden"—usually those high in fat or sugar. If they eat a forbidden food they break a psychological rule, which often leads them to decide that, since it is broken anyway, the diet may as well be forgotten until the next day, when it can be started afresh. Breaking a diet rule can also contribute to a cycle of perceived failure, which in turn leads to a loss of self-esteem and a comfort-eating response. Dieting itself can therefore contribute to the cycle of anxiety and overeating.

It can be very helpful to analyze your emotional state in relation to your food intake. Keeping a diary, for example, of what you ate and how you felt at the time may help you to pinpoint any emotional issues that need to be confronted. For instance, did you eat a large number of cookies while thinking about a relationship problem? Once you have established a link it is important to take steps to address the emotional problem. In the case of serious anxiety or depression, consulting a counselor may often be the best solution.

THE PSYCHOLOGY OF WEIGHT
For many people, body image becomes an obsession: impossible goals are set that can never be fulfilled. This leads to frustration

and depression at perceived failure. It is important to realize that your self-image is profoundly influenced by factors over which you have little control. Advertising images, models in magazines and on billboards, film and television stars—all embody ideals of beauty that most people find impossible to attain. However unrealistic we know these ideals to be, it's difficult to be immune to such influences at a subconscious level.

There has been a great deal of research on the topic of body image and how women, in particular, often take an exaggeratedly negative view of their own bodies. Studies have shown that, in general, men have a more accurate assessment and acceptance of their body shapes. It is also interesting to note that a woman's perception of the most desirable female figure tends to be significantly thinner than the most desirable figure nominated by men, and more importantly, it is thinner than most doctors would recommend for optimal health.

Because some women so rigidly apply society's "thin" messages to themselves, their self-esteem becomes almost entirely based on their body size and shape, and this increases their risk of developing eating disorders. In order to achieve realistic weight goals it is necessary to establish or to reclaim a sense of oneself as an individual and not as a reflection of the norms that society's current fashion dictates.

EATING DISORDERS

Two extreme and well-known examples of abnormal eating behavior are anorexia nervosa and bulimia (see page 37). Both these disorders involve an over-concern with weight and shape and an obsessive effort to continually lose weight, either by not eating or by indulging in inappropriate responses to food such as vomiting or using laxatives. The reasons that a distorted image develops are complex (see below), but some psychologists believe that part of the blame lies with the unrealistic images of beautiful women that bombard the public today. These can have a strong effect on impressionable teenage girls or young women, who comprise more than 90 percent of eating disorder cases. Boys are affected only occasionally.

Anorexia nervosa is characterized by severe weight loss, to the extent that a woman's periods stop (they return once normal weight is regained). Other health risks include malnutrition, an increased risk of fracture due to osteoporosis, and, in extreme cases, death from starvation. Metabolic and other changes brought about by their erratic eating behavior also increases their risk of

continued on page 42

Dangerous ideals
In 1995 the trend for extremely thin models went too far for a major watch manufacturer. The company threatened to suspend advertising from a top-selling British fashion magazine in response to its use of such models. One of the young women, with a height of 1.75 m (5 ft, 9 in), weighed only 48 kg (106 lb).

WHAT CAUSES EATING DISORDERS?

Eating disorders such as anorexia nervosa and bulimia are the result of complex and poorly understood causes. Sexual and mental abuse, parental conflict, pressure from sports coaches, and the influence of society's ideals of body shape have all been implicated. As shown in the summary below, sufferers fall into a cycle of depression and low self-esteem, which they express through an obsession with their weight. Once they start to link body image and eating with mood and self-esteem, a pattern of extreme dieting and/or bingeing and subsequent self-loathing can result. They may see weight loss as the solution to their problems and feel that exerting strict control over their diet will help them control their emotional difficulties. All eating disorders are potentially dangerous. Sufferers are unlikely to help themselves and often deny having a problem. It is very important to break this negative cycle; usually professional help is needed.

DISTORTED PERCEPTION
Social pressures and emotional problems can make a person of normal body weight perceive herself as overweight.

Stress, depression, low self-esteem. Morbid obsession with fatness.	Severe dieting. Overactivity. Obsession with exercise.	Severe weight loss. Fatigue, weakness. Poor skin and hair. Continued obsession with weight.	Uncontrolled binge eating followed by induced vomiting.	Severe psychological disorders for which professional advice is needed.

Clinical Psychologist

Clinical psychologists treat a range of disorders, including eating problems. They also deal with psychiatric depression, anxiety and behavioral disorders, and some severe mental illnesses such as schizophrenia and manic depression.

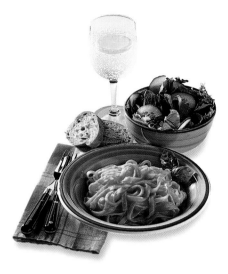

REGULATING EATING PATTERNS
Because people with eating disorders often skip meals and then end up bingeing later due to hunger, eating regular meals can be the first step on the road to recovery. Meals should be of moderate size and healthy content, so that they do not prompt any after-eating guilt responses.

Clinical psychologists may train in several areas of psychology, including psychotherapy. Their aim is to help people find their own solutions to problems such as binge eating, relationship difficulties, or phobias. They are essentially concerned with a patient's current situation, but may ask about problems in the past if this seems relevant to the person's behavior. Their questions seek to uncover what patients think about themselves, their problems, and goals. When treatment is aimed at changing the way they think in order to correct self-defeating behavior, this is termed cognitive therapy. When the focus is on correcting faulty habits, it is called behavior modification. Some psychologists combine the two approaches.

THE TRUE PICTURE
People with eating disorders often see a distorted picture of their own body shape. A clinical psychologist can help a patient recognize the truth about her image, which is an important part of recovery.

What is the difference between a clinical psychologist and a psychiatrist?

A clinical psychologist is someone who has been trained in a number of psychological techniques that have practical applications for different psychological problems. Most have doctorate degrees in psychology and in many states must meet certain requirements for licensing, but they cannot prescribe drugs unless they have a medical degree.

A psychiatrist first obtains a medical degree and then specializes in psychiatric disorders, often treating them with drugs. For eating disorders, however, psychological treatments are usually more effective than medications. Thus, there is likely to be little difference in the treatment offered by clinical psychologists and psychiatrists in practice, although a psychiatrist still has the option of prescribing drugs if they are necessary.

Do I need a referral from my primary-care physician?

This is the usual route. Although other health professionals, for example, dietitians or counselors, can make the recommendation, under most insurance plans in the United States, a primary-care physician must make the referral. If you feel unable to talk to your doctor, or if he or she is reluctant to refer you to a psychologist without a satisfactory explanation, then consider finding another physician who can help.

What will I need to talk to the psychologist about?

This question is difficult to answer in general terms, as it depends on the specific treatment you are seeking. When treatment is based on cognitive or behavioral therapy or a combination of the two (see box, far right), a psychologist will generally want to know about your eating habits and your thoughts about weight and shape. You may be asked to complete some homework tasks, such as keeping a food diary or writing a list of arguments for and against regaining control of eating habits. Problems other than an eating disorder, for example, relationship difficulties, may also be relevant.

Some therapists will ask about problems you might have had as a child and aim to resolve these as part of the overall treatment. It is up to you how much you tell the psychologist. You should remember, though, that this person is there to help, and, if you are not honest, he or she will have an incomplete picture of your problem and may not be able to help as effectively.

How long will I need to see a therapist and how often?

A general course of treatment is usually between 16 and 20 sessions. More or fewer may be recommended, depending on how severe your problem is. Initially, you may be asked to attend a couple of times a week. Later sessions may be spaced farther apart. The frequency of sessions will be negotiated between you and the psychologist. If you have not improved significantly within the initial course of treatment, you may be offered more sessions.

Will I need to see anyone else during treatment?

This depends on the nature of your problem and the resources available. Options include a dietitian to help devise a sensible eating plan, family therapy if you are young and still live at home with your parents, or even group therapy with other people who suffer from similar problems.

Irrespective of the facilities available, your doctor may be kept informed by your psychologist, so that he or she can offer additional support or medical help.

Origins

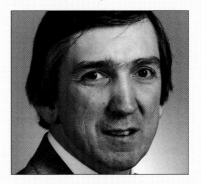

Professor Christopher Fairburn at Oxford University has led the development of two treatments for bulimia—cognitive-behavioral therapy, or CBT, and interpersonal therapy, or IPT. The one most widely used is CBT. It aims to alter the negative thoughts that contribute to bulimia and help a patient regain control over eating while modifying concerns about weight, shape, and dieting. Many bulimia sufferers have problematic relationships with parents or partners, and IPT focuses largely on these issues.

WHAT YOU CAN DO AT HOME

Here are two self-help methods you can try in conjunction with your professional treatment to help relieve your worries between sessions:

▶ *Try to limit weighing yourself to once a day, always at the same time. Work up to once a week. People with eating disorders often weigh themselves constantly. But because weight can fluctuate naturally by a pound or two every day because of changes in fluid retention, this fluctuation should not be taken to indicate long-term weight gain. As your eating patterns normalize, you are likely to find that your weight also stabilizes, though day-to-day fluctuations will probably continue.*

▶ *To increase both your motivation and optimism, write two letters as if it were five years in the future. Each letter could be to yourself, a friend (but do not send*

it), or someone imaginary. In the first letter, write as if you still have the eating problems. Set down how you feel, what life with the eating disorder has been like over the past five years, and the effects on your self-esteem, your health, and your relationships. In the second letter, write as if you have recovered completely. Describe how you feel now. Acknowledge how difficult the process has been but also relate the benefits that have resulted from recovery, such as improvements in your lifestyle and relationships. These letters should be as detailed and personal as possible.

WRITING RELIEF
Writing a letter can allow you to release your true feelings. It will focus your mind on your problem and boost your motivation by helping you envisage success.

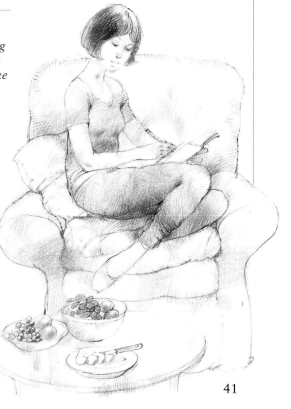

heart disease. Anorectics are often very secretive about their dietary habits, making treatment difficult.

It can be less easy to identify those suffering from bulimia because they tend to be of normal weight. Bulimics have periodic uncontrollable binges, which are usually followed by self-induced vomiting, abuse of laxatives or diuretics, fasting, obsessive exercising, and taking such drugs as diet pills and amphetamines in an attempt to avoid weight gain. The health risks of bulimia, although generally less severe than those of anorexia, are nevertheless serious. They include dehydration and loss of potassium, which causes weakness and cramps. The gastric acid in vomit may also damage teeth and the lining of the throat.

Causes of anorexia and bulimia

Anorexia nervosa has been recognized for centuries, but bulimia was first described in 1979 by Professor Gerald Russell, then at the Institute of Psychiatry in London. It is hotly debated whether the number of women with anorexia has increased over the years but it is almost universally accepted that the numbers of women with bulimia

has increased since the 1960s, with the rise of the diet culture, and women with bulimia now far outnumber those with anorexia.

Some people blame today's image of the supermodel and the craze for waif-like female bodies for eating disorders. Whether or not these accusations are just—and the extent to which weight-reducing diets encourage eating disorders is unknown—these are certainly not the only causes. There are many other possible factors. They can include emotional difficulties during childhood, sexual abuse, a difficult relationship with parents, and neglect, as well as problems that arise during adulthood, including low self-esteem, emotional and relationship problems, and a fear of sex. Some research suggests that eating disorders stem in part from brain chemical and hormonal imbalances.

Few women develop bulimia in its most severe form, which lies at the far end of the spectrum of eating problems. However, minor eating disorders can eventually lead to bulimia if the psychological problems behind them are not fully addressed, and many women show some signs of bulimia, but at a much less severe level.

THE HEALTH RISKS LINKED TO ANOREXIA NERVOSA

Once body weight drops to a third or more below normal, signs of malnutrition such as a gaunt, emaciated appearance become evident. The normal hormonal balance is disturbed, leading to thinning hair, bone wasting, and an absence of periods. Poor vitamin and mineral intake causes deficiency disorders and disrupts the immune system, increasing risk of disease. Lack of body fat leads to rapid loss of body heat, sometimes to a life-threatening degree.

Hair gets thinner as a result of hormone changes and a lack of nutrients. At the same time, a fine downy hair (lanugo) may grow on the body.

Breasts revert to prepubescent size because of muscle wasting, loss of body fat, and hormone changes.

Ovaries are affected by hormone imbalances, leading to cessation of periods (amenorrhea) and infertility.

Skin is very dry and nails are fragile because of disrupted hormone levels and poor diet.

Bones become brittle and fracture easily (osteoporosis), as a result of reduced calcium intake and hormone imbalances.

Teeth are gradually worn away by repeated self-induced vomiting, which causes decay, tooth loss, and degeneration of the jawbone.

Heart tissue is damaged by the low dietary intake of protein, vitamins, and minerals, leading to irregular heartbeat and other cardiac disorders.

Kidney damage and the risk of kidney failure result from long-term malnutrition.

Muscle wasting occurs as muscles are broken down to provide vital energy in order to compensate for low calorie intake.

Intestines suffer long-term disruption to their digestive functions because of a lack of vital nutrients.

LIFESTYLE FACTORS

Changes in the way we live are emerging as the most significant reasons for the general increase in obesity in Western society over the past few decades.

Factors such as where, how, and what we eat, combined with a decline in physical activity, have significantly affected the average weight of populations in North America. In order to bring about a weight change it is necessary to resist the influences of society and, in some cases, change one's lifestyle toward healthier day-to-day living. The rate of increase in obesity in Western society is far too rapid to be accounted for by genetic factors alone. In the United States, for example, at least one person in three is on a weight-loss diet at any given time and, despite these efforts to reduce, the numbers remain constant. Nearly 90 percent of dieters regain within five years all or most of any weight lost.

LIFESTYLE AND WEIGHT

It is only over the last 50 years that people have had almost unlimited access to cheap calorie-dense food. Both take-out food outlets and frozen or canned convenience foods from supermarkets have had a dramatic influence on the diet of the general population. These foods tend to be high in fat, contributing to an overall calorie increase. The ease with which such foods can be bought and consumed has also encouraged the development of a "snacking" culture where, rather than eating regular balanced meals, many people snack on nutritionally poor convenience foods. The fact that children indulge in regular snacking is particularly worrying, when as much as 45 percent of their energy requirements may be met by such high-fat foods as pizza, chips, hot dogs, and ice cream.

At the same time that dietary habits have changed, physical activity has declined. The use of automobiles has increased and the technological revolution has outmoded many physically demanding jobs. Manual labor inside and outside the home has also declined. Leisure pursuits have become more sedentary, with television watching now the most popular pastime for many people. The change in health and fitness of the general population was highlighted in 1996, when the British army announced that its young recruits were failing fitness tests passed by earlier generations.

The effects of affluence

Like many chronic conditions, obesity appears to be more common among the poorer people of developed countries, which suggests it relates to lifestyle factors. There is a strong correlation between social class and inactivity, and the relationship is stronger than that between social class and the amount of energy-foods eaten or the amount of fat consumed. While wealthier people often take more expensive steps toward improving their health and fitness, such as enrolling at a gym, poor people tend to remain home-bound, particularly when they have young children, and television watching and similarly sedentary pursuits are often their primary leisure activities.

In developing countries the reverse is true. Individuals seem to be at higher risk of becoming obese the wealthier they become. This is probably due to a combination of

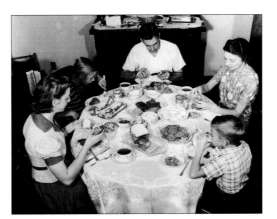

A FAMILY AFFAIR
One drawback to modern living is that families do not dine together as often as they used to.

factors, such as a reduction in exercise and the change to a higher-calorie diet, as they embrace the lifestyle of an affluent society. The same is also true of migrant workers who move to more affluent countries; for example, Indian immigrants to the United Kingdom and Canada.

Extensive entertaining and socializing also tend to be features of affluent societies. Eating out while on a weight-control plan can be a problem, because many restaurants don't offer alternatives to their rich, exotic foods; add to this the temptations of desserts and alcohol, and the goal of controlled, healthy eating becomes difficult to achieve. But there are steps that can be taken to manage the situation (see right).

Alcohol is not only high in calories, it also reduces willpower. This means that after a few drinks it is easy to forget your good intentions and eat more than you originally intended. Moreover, alcohol is an appetite stimulant, so you are likely to eat more than usual if alcohol is served with your meal. Parties and pub or club nights can also be a problem because you are likely to be tempted to snack on calorie-laden, high-fat foods such as nuts and chips.

Examining your lifestyle and quantifying how much exercise you do in relation to the amount and type of food you eat can be a sobering experience. It might prompt you to find ways of introducing more activity into your daily routine. Walking to the store rather than taking the car, for example, could be a first step toward a more active life.

HEALTHIER SOCIAL EATING AND DRINKING

Going out for dinner needn't spell doom for your diet, and you don't have to avoid social events when trying to control your weight. These simple techniques can help you eat healthily.

▶ *Eat something nutritious and filling such as pasta and a salad before going out to a party or for drinks. This will reduce the temptation to snack on unhealthy treats at the function and will give you energy to enjoy yourself.*

▶ *Choose restaurants that have low-fat, nutritious options on their menus. Remember, too, you can always ask the waiter for advice. Any food that is broiled, grilled, or steamed is a good choice. You can also reduce the fat in a meal by removing the skin from chicken or trimming fat from meat.*

▶ *Drink water some of the time while at a bar or a party. This not only will help you control your alcohol intake, but also will reduce such negative effects of alcohol as dehydration.*

THE ROLE OF STRESS

Some stress can be beneficial when facing challenges; for example, a special project at work might be achieved more successfully with the help of a little stress, because in small amounts it helps to focus the mind. However, too much stress can damage health in the long-term, as it can reduce the efficiency of the immune system and lead to fatigue and illness.

Whether the physiological response to daily stress has any relation to weight itself still remains unknown. In some cases, stress actually increases metabolism, because adrenaline raises the body's heart rate. Digestive problems, often a symptom of stress, can lead to loss of appetite, thus causing some people to lose weight as their appetite decreases. For others, the opposite may occur, as comfort eating is a common response to stress, and weight gain results.

In either case, erratic eating behavior, such as skipping meals or bingeing, tends to lead to eventual weight gain. Reducing daily stress can therefore be helpful in controlling weight. Regular exercise is a useful stress reliever, as are relaxation techniques such as meditation and visualization.

NUTRITIONAL VALUES OF SOME FAST FOODS

Many fast foods are high in fat (therefore delivering a lot of energy), yet offer insubstantial nutritional value. Although high-fat foods do fill you up, you tend to feel hunger pangs and a drive to eat sooner after eating them than if you had eaten foods that are high in protein, carbohydrates, and fiber.

FOOD	CALORIES	FAT (g)	CHOLESTEROL (mg)
Bacon and egg sandwich	427	22.7 g	246 mg
2 pieces extra crispy chicken	544	37 g	168 mg
Cola, 350 ml (12 fl oz)	136	0 g	0 mg
Quarter-pound burger	193	12.2 g	61 mg
Cheese and tomato pizza slice	235	11.8 g	16 mg
Milk shake, 350 ml (12 fl oz)	444	14 g	42 mg
French fries, regular size	280	15.5 g	0 mg

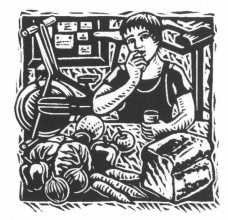

CHAPTER 3

MAINTAINING A HEALTHY WEIGHT

Controlling your weight can be a lot easier to manage if you understand why you feel the urge to eat. This chapter explains what your basic nutritional needs are, how to distinguish between hunger and appetite, and how to handle the physiological and lifestyle changes that affect your weight from childhood through old age.

WHY WE EAT

Fuel is vital for our survival, for good health, and for efficient functioning of the body. In modern Western society, however, we often turn to food for reasons other than true hunger.

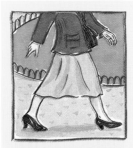

QUICK FITNESS TIP
If possible, walk part of the way to and from work. Alternatively, go for a brisk 20-minute walk at lunchtime.

The body has mechanisms to ensure an adequate intake of food (see page 28), but there are many other factors that urge you to eat. Close-ups of food on television can stimulate your appetite; you might be bored or unhappy and use food as a comfort or a diversion; or you may be tempted to overeat at a dinner party.

FEELING HUNGRY

Hunger is the physiological need for food—the body's innate response to variations in its food supply. The body provides clear messages when it needs food: your stomach contracts producing a "rumble;" in extreme cases you may feel weak and faint. Appetite is the desire for food—a learned response to sensations or thoughts associated with eating. It produces several physical effects, including increased salivation and secretion of digestive juices in the stomach. An initial step in a weight-loss program is to recognize the difference between these two states: to separate an urge for food from a need. Many things can make you feel hungry by sensually or psychologically stimulating your appetite. However, this does not mean that you are physically in need of food.

SOCIAL ENVIRONMENT

Food is one of the things that binds members of a society, and in most cultures eating is among the most important of social acts. All the major holidays and celebrations incorporate food as either the central celebration (for example, the Christmas Day feast), or as an important part of the festivities—the wedding or birthday cake, for instance. Relationships are cemented by food. Loved ones are taken out to dinner and lovers even feed one another as a sign of their affection. Friends meet over dinner and drinks and, in this context, refusing food or alcohol can be interpreted as a snub. Business relationships are also strengthened by sharing food; weight is often a problem

FOOD FOR FEASTS AND FESTIVALS

Food has a spiritual importance in many faiths. Hindus, for example, worship the cow, and so hold butter and milk to be sacred. They also revere coconut because they believe its three "eyes" symbolize their god Shiva. In Jewish tradition the house must be cleared of all leavened bread, which is made with yeast, before the Passover feast is celebrated. This festival marks the Israelites' escape from slavery in Egypt, during which they were unable to prepare leavened bread because they could not wait for dough to rise. Unleavened matzo bread is eaten during Passover and is broken in two to symbolize Moses' parting of the Red Sea.

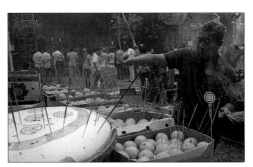

GIFTS FOR THE GHOSTS
During the Hungry Ghosts Festival, held in Hong Kong from mid-August to mid-September, food and other gifts are offered in order to placate restless spirits who might otherwise take revenge on the living.

for a sales representative or self-employed business person who dines with clients to help build a trusting working relationship.

In any social environment we may feel pressure to eat more than we actually want or need in order to smooth interaction or foster a sense of camaraderie and goodwill. If you have identified a link between overeating and social gatherings, however, you can start to make changes. Schedule fewer meetings—work or social—around mealtimes and suggest other activities for occasions when you meet friends, such as going for a walk or playing tennis.

EMOTIONAL GRATIFICATION

We also eat for more complex emotional reasons (see page 36). We may eat because we are unhappy or depressed, because we're bored, or because we're stressed. Feeling full can be warm and reassuring. A study of foreign students learning English in London in 1985 showed that feelings of homesickness lessened considerably while they were eating and immediately afterward.

Other studies have shown that people who have been traumatized as children often turn to food for comfort and nurturing. These childhood habits can sometimes foster a weight problem in adulthood. Comfort eating occurs in many different situations—at home, at work, at social gatherings, for example—and for a variety of reasons—boredom, disappointment, dissatisfaction, loneliness, unhappiness, anger, or lack of confidence. Establishing how your emotions influence your eating patterns is crucial in maintaining healthy weight.

EATING FOR THE RIGHT REASONS

A weight-loss diet will usually fail if food is used for comfort or as a diversion from other problems, but there are ways to minimize these impulses. To begin, you need to write down in a diary the exact details of what you currently eat. Include hidden foodstuffs such as the mayonnaise in a salad and be scrupulously honest about between-meal snacks.

As well as writing down exactly what you ate, make a note of how you felt at the time. Were you unhappy or bored? And did this coincide with eating more cookies than intended while watching television? Keeping this kind of diary will not only make you far more aware of exactly how much you really

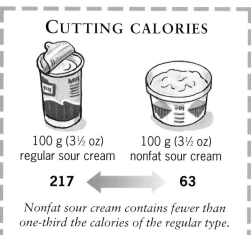

CUTTING CALORIES

100 g (3½ oz) regular sour cream

100 g (3½ oz) nonfat sour cream

217 ← **63**

Nonfat sour cream contains fewer than one-third the calories of the regular type.

consume during the day, it may also help you establish if there is a pattern to your eating, so that you can recognize any danger signs.

Your diary may reveal a few surprises. Research carried out in the UK in 1986 showed that obese women underestimated their food intake by an average of 800 calories a day. Another study in Holland, done in 1988and involving 525 men, revealed that the most overweight individuals displayed the biggest discrepancy between actual calories consumed and estimated intake.

If your diary shows a link between boredom and snacking, in the first instance you will probably need to make sure that you have low-calorie snacks on hand such as fruit or rice cakes. In the longer term you should look at why you are feeling bored

BURNING OFF CALORIES: *Walking*

Walking is an ideal exercise for all ages. It is a good alternative to jogging, helping to develop cardiovascular fitness with far less risk of injury. For maximum aerobic benefit, maintain a brisk pace.

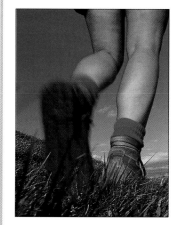

Muscle groups benefiting
Regular walking will firm up all the leg muscles, especially those in the thighs and calves.

Equipment
Thick socks and a sturdy pair of walking shoes with good ankle support will help guard against blisters and sprains.

Calories burned
At 3 miles per hour, you burn 5 calories per minute: that's 300 calories per hour.

and what you can do to change You could, for example, join an evening class after work instead of watching television.

Eating while watching television may also distract you from realizing how much food you are consuming and prevent you from giving your food due appreciation. Sitting down to a meal at the table and eating slowly so that you savor the food you have prepared will help you feel more satisfied and properly fed, and may prevent snacking later in the evening.

Think about any habits that you connect automatically, such as sofa/video/cookies; cold/comfort/hot chocolate; work/coffee/doughnut. Interrupt them with healthier alternatives, for example, sofa/video/fruit; cold/comfort/herbal tea; work/coffee/cereal bar. This has the effect of questioning your choice of foods while making beneficial changes to your existing behavior patterns.

Avoid food shopping on an empty stomach, and before any item goes into the cart, ask yourself whether you really need it.

Some people find that it helps to make a list—and stick to it. Before mealtimes you should also think about each food item you are planning to eat and decide if it is really necessary and whether there is a healthier alternative, such as one that is lower in fat.

Instead of comfort eating, look for an alternative treat such as a long soak in the bath, a home manicure or pedicure, booking a free makeover session, or buying a bunch of flowers. Going for a long walk, especially in picturesque surroundings, can also be distracting.

If your cravings for food become very strong, try to keep yourself busy. Clean out a cupboard, for instance, or reorganize your book, music, or video collection; put on a favorite piece of music or look at photographs that evoke happy memories. Write a letter to a friend you have not seen or spoken to for a long time or phone someone for a chat. You could also tidy up your wardrobe and mix and match your clothes to create new outfits.

THE HUNGER GAUGE

Rediscovering eating as a response to feeling hungry, and being more objective about how hungry you actually are when you eat, can be a major step on the way to successful long-term weight control. The hunger gauge below aims to help you measure how hungry you are. It is best to eat when you are only moderately hungry and to stop eating when you feel satisfied but could eat a little more. Your food intake should adequately sustain you during the day, so that from one meal to the next you do not become ravenously hungry. If you eat at level 1 when you are desperately hungry, you are at risk of overeating.

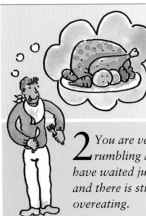

1 *You are desperately hungry and experiencing clear physical signs of hunger such as feeling faint and shaky. There is a risk of bingeing once you start to eat.*

2 *You are very hungry—your stomach is rumbling and you feel a little tired. You have waited just a little too long before eating, and there is still a risk of overeating.*

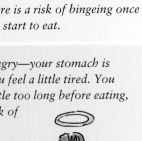

3 *You are moderately hungry; you have an appetite for food and a pleasant sense of anticipation . This is the ideal time to start eating. Eat until you are satisfied and no more.*

4 *You feel satisfied. You could perhaps be tempted to eat dessert, but it's not essential. This is the ideal time to stop; aim to leave the table wanting just a little more and you will avoid feeling overly full.*

5 *You are too full. You left the table a little late, because you could not resist the temptation of another small helping, and now you feel uncomfortable.*

6 *You are very full. You ignored all the signs to stop eating and now feel weighed down. You may also be experiencing indigestion or heartburn.*

WHAT TO EAT TO STAY HEALTHY

The main purpose of eating is to provide the right fuel for your body to perform efficiently. Even when trying to lose weight, you should still be eating a healthful balance of foods.

Getting to know your nutritional needs, the roles of different food groups, and what constitutes a well-balanced diet makes good sense for your health.

A BALANCING ACT

The principle of healthy eating is balance: consuming the right amounts of carbohydrate, protein, and fat from a variety of foods that also provide essential vitamins and minerals, and taking in the right amount of energy (calories) to equal what you burn up. Complex carbohydrates—such as bread, pasta, rice, and potatoes—should make up the largest part of your diet. The next largest source of food should be fruits and vegetables. Meat and dairy products are important for protein, but are needed only in modest amounts. Foods high in fats and sugars, such as cookies, pies, cakes, and chocolate, should be eaten sparingly .

The chart below shows about how many calories are needed each day for adults, according to body weight and activity. You can roughly calculate your own requirements as follows. **Basic needs,** allow 10 calories per pound. **Normal activities,** allow 3 calories per pound of body weight plus extra calories used for exercise. **Adjustment for age,** subtract 2 percent of total calories for each decade after age 30. Example: If you are a 60-year-old woman who weighs 130 pounds and walks 3 miles each day: basic needs, 10 x 130 = **1,300**; normal activities, 3 x 130 = **390**; 3-mile walk, 3 x 100 = **300**; total calories = **1990**; age adjustment, .06 x 1990 = **119**. Total calories needed per day = **1871**.

continued on page 52

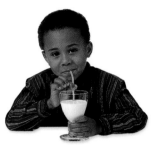

FOOD FOR GROWTH
Milk provides a rich source of both protein and calcium. Most nutritionists recommend that children drink whole milk up to the age of five, because they need the extra energy provided by the fat.

UNDERSTANDING YOUR CALORIE NEEDS

To avoid putting on weight, it helps to know your daily caloric needs. This figure can be calculated according to your gender, weight, and level of activity. As shown below, the less active you are, the fewer calories you need, but as soon as you start to include a reasonable level of regular physical activity in your life, your energy requirements rise. Remember that needs will be lower during periods of inactivity, and you should reduce your calorie intake accordingly.

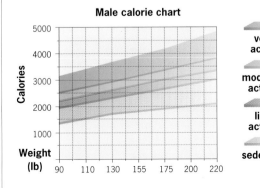

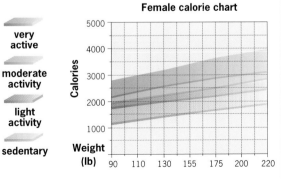

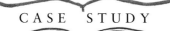

The Overworked Manager

Leading a stressful, busy life in the fast lane can lead to unhealthy lifestyle habits, such as eating high-fat foods, exercising infrequently or not at all, and smoking. In the long term, these habits can produce potentially serious health problems. It is important to recognize what is happening and take the necessary steps to prevent further damage.

Andrew is a 44-year-old account manager who is married with two children. He has smoked an average of 20 cigarettes a day since his teens and now becomes breathless going up stairs. He does no exercise other than taking his children to the park, and then only as often as his job permits. He is overweight, which he attributes to regular client entertaining. His work is pressured, and he arrives home late almost every night. He looks in on the children, has dinner (with wine), and then does his paperwork for the next day. In the morning he has coffee and leaves for work very early. His father died at 55 from a heart attack, as did his grandfather, but Andrew feels he has no time to do anything about his lifestyle.

WHAT SHOULD ANDREW DO?

Andrew needs to recognize that his lifestyle and genetic inheritance make him susceptible to heart disease. He has to take steps to improve his lifestyle, starting with giving up smoking. He can delegate responsibilities and prioritize his time to ease pressures at work, so he will have more time to spend with his family and in doing exercise. When dining with clients he can select lower-fat alternatives from menus and cut back on his alcohol intake. These measures will not only reduce calories and improve his health but also sharpen his perfor-mance at work. Walking the children to school in the morning would better family relationships, and the exercise could help relieve his stress.

Action Plan

EATING HABITS
Cut back on the amount of alcohol consumption and high-fat foods in the diet to reduce overall calorie intake.

FITNESS
Incorporate regular exercise into the daily routine to improve fitness, relieve stress, and burn up excess calories.

WORK
Delegate work whenever possible, and prioritize the workload to allow adequate time for personal health and family commitments.

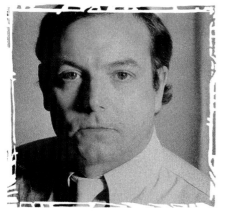

FITNESS
Busy people find it hard to make time for exercise during the day.

WORK
A demanding job places physical and emotional pressures on people.

EATING HABITS
A high-fat diet can cause high cholesterol and damage the arteries. High alcohol consumption increases the risk of heart disease and hypertension.

HOW THINGS TURNED OUT FOR ANDREW

Andrew cut back his cigarettes and during working lunches chose low-fat options and soft drinks. He gave his staff more responsibility, which alleviated some of his pressure and made him more effective at work. These changes meant he could leave later in the morning and walk his children to school. As family relationships improved, he spent more time with the children on weekends, going for bicycle rides regularly. In three months he had reduced his weight by 6.3 kg (14 lb).

WHAT MAKES A HEALTHY DIET?

There are seven essential nutrients that sustain human life: water, protein, carbohydrates, fat, vitamins, minerals, and fiber. A healthy diet should include a balanced intake of all of these. Both excesses and deficiencies can be harmful to the body's health and efficiency. For example, not eating enough fruit and vegetables can lead to a weakening of the body's immune system. Food elements also interact; many people are not aware, for example, that excess protein can deplete calcium levels in the body. To keep your weight under control, look for foods that deliver relatively little fat but provide other essential nutrients.

Water is the body's most basic need. It is required for almost every function, and without it you would die in just a few days. It is important not to ignore thirst. Some people try to lose weight by reducing fluid intake, but this is dangerous. As a general guide you should drink eight glasses of water daily. The body also obtains water from food: milk, eggs, meat, vegetables, and fruit all have a high water content.

Protein, made up of amino acids, is essential for the growth and maintenance of body tissue, blood cells, hormones, and enzymes. The best sources of protein are meat, poultry, fish, milk products, and eggs. Vegetables, grains, fruits, legumes, seeds, and nuts contain lesser amounts. Ten to 15 percent of your daily calorie intake should be from protein.

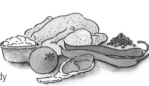

Carbohydrates provide fuel to meet energy needs. Complex carbohydrates, or starches, are found in many plant foods such as grains, potatoes, and rice. Simple carbohydrates are prevalent in fruit. Carbohydrates should form 55 to 60 percent of your diet.

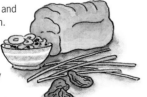

Fiber is indigestible carbohydrate and is very important for general health. There are two types, insoluble and soluble. Insoluble fiber aids in the digestive process; it can help prevent hemorrhoids and may also protect against cancer of the lower bowel. Sources include brown rice, bran, whole-grain cereals, and broccoli. Soluble fiber is thought to help reduce cholesterol and thus reduce the risk of heart and arterial disease. It is found in oats, peas, beans, root vegetables, and citrus fruits. Recommended intake of fiber is 20g to 35 g per day from different sources.

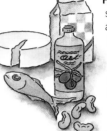

Fat is essential as an energy store, to insulate the body against rapid heat loss, help produce hormones, cushion vital organs such as the liver and kidneys, and aid in the absorption of certain vitamins. Fat should represent no more 30 percent of the diet, but many people eat more. There are two main types of fats: saturated (prevalent in meat, poultry, and whole-milk products) and unsaturated (the predominant fat in vegetable oils). Fried and sugary foods that are high in saturated fat should be avoided, as they offer little nutritional value. On the other hand, unsaturated fats, especially the monounsaturated fat in olive oil, may help protect against heart disease.

Vitamins are organic compounds, essential for bodily growth, function, maintenance, and repair. They are categorized into two groups, water soluble and fat soluble. Water soluble vitamins, including the B complex group and vitamin C, need to be replenished daily because they are not stored in the body's tissues. Fat soluble vitamins, including A, D, E, and K, are stored by the body for long periods of time, and so excessive intake may be harmful. A balanced diet that includes plenty of fresh fruit and vegetables and cereals should provide all the vitamins that the body needs.

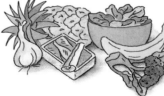

Minerals are essential inorganic compounds that aid energy production and body maintenance as well as assisting in the control of body reactions and reflexes. There are three groups; macrominerals, electrolytes (a subgroup of macrominerals), and micro, or trace, elements. The macrominerals, calcium, magnesium, and phosphorus, and the electrolytes, chloride, potassium, and sodium , are required in larger amounts. The body needs trace minerals—chromium, copper, fluoride, iodine, iron, manganese, molybdenum, selenium, sulfur, and zinc—in minuscule amounts. A diet that includes a wide range of animal and plant foods should provide all the minerals essential for health.

A BALANCED DIET – AS EASY AS 12345

The 1+2+3+4+5 plan equals a balanced daily diet. Each day, eat 1 portion of meat, poultry, seafood or meat substitute, 2 portions of dairy products, 3 pieces of fruit, 4 portions of vegetables, 5 servings of bread/cereal, plus a small treat. This menu shows how you can spread these portions throughout your day.

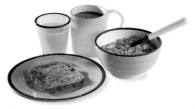

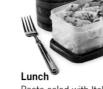

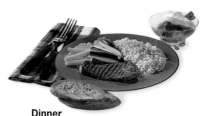

Breakfast
Muesli with low-fat or skim milk, orange juice, 1 slice whole-grain toast with low-fat margarine, coffee with low-fat or skim milk = 1 portion dairy, 2 portions bread/cereal, and 1 fruit.

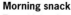

Morning snack
Tea with low-fat or skim milk, 1 banana = 1 piece fruit, 1/3 portion dairy. (The milk and yogurt for the snack and lunch combine to make 1 dairy portion.)

Lunch
Pasta salad with Italian green beans, corn, and yogurt dressing, coffee with low-fat or skim milk = 2/3 portion dairy, 1 portion bread/cereal, 2 portions vegetable.

Dinner
Grilled steak, brown rice, steamed zucchini and carrots, garlic bread, and trifle for dessert = 1 portion meat, 2 portions bread/cereal, 2 portions vegetable, and 1 treat.

Afternoon snack
1 apple = 1 piece fruit.

CHANGING NEEDS

During your lifetime there will be periods when nutritional and calorie requirements have to be adjusted or changed in response to different demands made upon your body.

Childhood

Infants and young children require energy for growth and so can eat more calorie-rich food than adults. Besides being more physically active in general, a child has a metabolic rate that is proportionally higher than an adult's, so energy is burned off much faster. Young children should eat larger amounts of dairy products than adults, since these are ideal sources of calcium and high-quality protein, both of which are essential for healthy growth. Children should never be put on a weight-loss plan without first consulting a doctor, because this can interfere with healthy growth.

DID YOU KNOW?

Protein is vital for growing children. Between the ages of 1 and 3 they need more than twice the amount of protein in relation to their size as an adult does. The amount required decreases as a child grows older, but children between 7 and 10 still need a third more total intake of protein in relation to their size than an adult.

Teenagers

Because the body undergoes a growth spurt at puberty, many teenagers—boys, in particular—are constantly hungry. A boy's basal metabolic rate (BMR) will remain high until around age 20, so he will be able to eat more food than an adult without putting on weight. A girl's BMR drops away much more quickly; by around age 15 it is generally at adult level. Neither adolescent boys nor girls should be encouraged to diet, as they still have relatively high nutritional needs. But there is a danger today that teenagers may exceed their energy needs and end up overweight because of the wide range of high-fat fast foods available to them. It is therefore important to encourage them to adopt healthy eating practices.

During and after pregnancy

Pregnancy and breast-feeding both place special dietary demands on the body. Foods that are rich in iron and calcium should be increased in the diet; iron can help prevent birth defects and calcium will be needed for the baby's bone development. Additional protein is also needed for the healthful development of the fetus.

Many women date the start of weight problems to pregnancy, but research shows that it is not because their metabolism has become sluggish after giving birth. Changes in lifestyle that follow childbirth, such as eating more (especially snacks) and being less active, are likely causes of weight gain or the reason that weight gained during pregnancy is not lost. This can be overcome by exercise and by making dietary changes. Breast feeding may help a woman lose this excess weight if it is continued for at least six months; it also supplies the best source of nutrition for the baby.

Old age

While the elderly should continue to follow recommended adult guidelines for nutrition, particular health problems associated with aging may be prevented or relieved by diet. Maintaining the recommended intake of calcium and vitamin D will protect against osteoporosis. Iron, from red meat, cereals, vegetables, and dried fruits, will be beneficial, as anemia can be a problem in old age, Also, increasing the amount of fiber will reduce constipation and help maintain a healthy digestive tract. Unless an elderly person remains particularly active, he or she will not need as many calories as someone in their 30s, and reducing overall intake of fat is a wise precaution against heart disease and other problems associated with fat.

SMOKING AND ALCOHOL

Smoking and excessive drinking can deplete your body of essential nutrients. Heavy drinkers often suffer from nutritional deficiencies because their dependence on alcohol causes them to neglect their diets. Also, excessive alcohol can interfere with metabolism of glucose, vitamins, and minerals.

CUTTING CALORIES

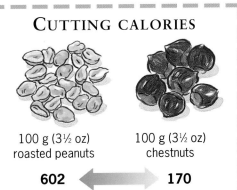

100 g (3½ oz) roasted peanuts | 100 g (3½ oz) chestnuts

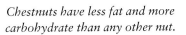

602 ⬅➡ **170**

Chestnuts have less fat and more carbohydrate than any other nut.

General recommendations in regard to alcohol is that it should be limited to one drink—a 4-ounce glass of wine, 1½ ounces of 80-proof liquor, or 12 ounces of beer—or two per day. If you drink in excess of these levels you may be damaging your health.

Alcohol has a high calorie content (7 calories per gram). Because it is toxic and cannot be stored by the body, it is converted directly to energy (95 percent is absorbed into the bloodstream within an hour after ingestion) and used before dietary energy sources. This means that drinking encourages food to be stored as fat and hence can cause weight gain. Also, alcohol weakens willpower, causing people to forget their good intentions. Research shows that people eat more at meals consumed with alcohol than when it is absent. Any weight-management plan should aim to limit alcohol intake.

TIPS FOR REDUCING ALCOHOL INTAKE

Any weight-loss plan will benefit greatly from a reduction in alcohol intake. Here are some suggestions on how to achieve this:

▶ *Halve the money you take with you to a bar, so that you cannot succumb to temptation.*

▶ *Make each drink last at least twice as long as you usually do.*

▶ *Drink single measures of spirits, not doubles.*

▶ *At a meal where wine is in abundance, have a jug of water on the table. For each glass of wine have two of water.*

QUIT SMOKING AND AVOID WEIGHT GAIN

Everybody knows that smoking is bad for health, but many people fear that if they quit they will gain weight. Smoking raises your metabolism; when you stop, the energy you take in from food is burned less efficiently. Furthermore, instead of eating less, many people eat high-fat snacks to replace cigarettes, and weight gain results. This can be avoided with diet and lifestyle changes.

CAROTENE FOR HEALTH *Low levels of beta-carotene have been linked with increased risk of cancer, so answering a nicotine craving with a carrot makes good sense.*

▶ *Eat fewer fatty foods and replace them with filling ones like rice and pasta.*

▶ *To boost your well-being and make up for the drop in your metabolism when you give up smoking, begin an exercise regimen. This can be as simple as going for a brisk 30-minute walk each day.*

▶ *Begin an evening course or start a new hobby to help refocus your mind away from smoking and keep you busy at times when you might otherwise smoke.*

SUITABLE SNACKS *Vary your low-fat snacks. Try sticks of raw vegetables, fresh fruit, or a filling drink of fruit blended with low-fat yogurt.*

LIFELONG HEALTHY WEIGHT

Long-term successful management of weight means forming good habits early in life. Many studies show that childhood obesity can lead to a lifetime of weight problems.

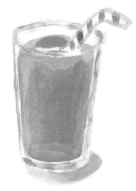

HOMEMADE FIZZ
Children love fizzy drinks but many canned drinks contain high amounts of sugar as well as other additives such as caffeine. A healthier option is to make your own fizzy drinks at home, using pure unsweetened fruit juice and carbonated water.

FAMILY OUTINGS
Days outdoors that focus on fun but are centered around exercise will improve the fitness of all the family. Bicycling trips in the countryside, long walks, or a day at a local swimming pool with wave machines and slides will all provide good aerobic exercise that is fun for the whole family.

There is strong evidence to show that an overweight child often grows up to be an overweight adult. One reason for this might be that eating the wrong types of food and doing insufficient exercise at a young age are difficult habits to break when you grow up.

CHILDREN'S WEIGHT
Alarmingly, the number of overweight and obese children is growing rapidly. The role of parents in promoting a healthy lifestyle is crucial. Statistics show that if a child has an obese parent he or she has a 40 percent chance of becoming obese also. The risk is doubled if both parents are fat.

When parents are uninformed or casual about healthy eating and they themselves do little exercise, they are introducing their children to lifestyle risks for obesity. Setting a good example by eating well is essential to teaching children a proper respect for their bodies. Using food as a way to control behavior can develop the wrong attitudes about diet in children. If sweets are given as

a reward for good behavior, and youngsters are told they must eat their vegetables in order to have dessert, messages are being sent about pleasant and unpleasant foods that can backfire at a later age. Sometimes problems arise, too, when young children are offered portions that are too large. A good rule of thumb for preschoolers is to put on the plate no more than one spoonful of each food for every year of age.

Being creative in meal planning can be a way to introduce healthier foods subtly into the family's diet. Most children enjoy the natural sweetness of fruit, and a fresh fruit salad served with low-fat yogurt is an appealing dessert. Disguising healthy food as fast food can also be successful: a hamburger made with lean meat that is grilled or broiled and served on a whole-grain bun with tomato and lettuce provides a healthy meal. It can also be helpful to gradually reduce the amount of salt and sugar added to recipes. Children will probably resist dramatic changes but may fail to notice a slow but steady decline.

Exercise needs to be introduced as an integral part of the family's lifestyle. Watching television and playing video or computer games should be balanced with more active pursuits. Many parents are anxious about their children playing unsupervised in parks and the streets, but some sociologists believe that increased levels of fear in our society have led to a cocooning mentality in which the home is considered the only safe place for children. Encouraging young people to join youth clubs and supervised sports activities can be a way to reduce this concern.

If children don't like sports (this can often be a problem with overweight or self-con-

continued on page 58

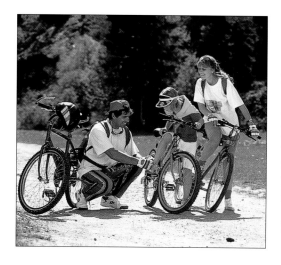

Middle-Age Spread

As people age their metabolism slows down and their body burns less energy. In addition, older people often live sedentary lives. But middle-age spread needn't be inevitable. Changing a diet to avoid fat and increasing levels of activity will both help to control weight. These changes will have positive benefits for health too, guarding against many diseases.

As you age your calorie requirements decline slightly because your resting metabolic rate decreases. Since fewer calories are burned, more will be stored as fat. Another effect of aging is that people become less active. The body tends to lose muscle and because muscle burns more energy than fat, this further reduces the body's energy needs. There are two ways of counterbalancing these effects. The first is to increase your exercise level so that your body stems the loss of muscle and burns more fat, and the second is to look at your diet and find ways of eating more healthily while decreasing the number of calories in the diet.

TIPS TO IMPROVE YOUR DIET

You can consume fewer calories without eating a smaller volume of food, if you choose lower fat items. You should also plan your eating to boost your metabolism. Don't skip meals, because this will cause your metabolism to be sluggish all day. Then, if you eat a large meal later to compensate, you cannot burn off all the extra calories consumed. Breakfast is especially important because it acts as a kick start to your metabolism, which slows during sleep.

▶ *Change to low-fat dairy alternatives.*
▶ *Use low-fat spreads instead of butter and cut back the amount you use.*
▶ *Choose lean cuts of meat. Trim off any visible fat. Remove the skin from poultry after cooking.*

COOKING BY STEAM
Steaming vegetables ensures that more vitamins are retained. Spread the raw vegetables out in the steamer so they cook evenly.

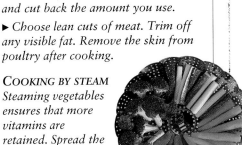

WARMING UP

Exercise has benefits for your general health, helping to maintain joint flexibility and mobility. It can also ease some of the symptoms of arthritis. Look at the type of exercise you are doing; if it is painful, there may be a better alternative. Swimming can be very beneficial, as it supports your weight while allowing freer movement of joints and muscles. Warming up is vital before more vigorous exercise, or it can be used as a daily routine to ease you from sedentary habits into an exercise regimen.

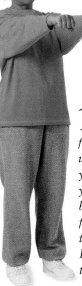

1 Arm swings. Stand with feet shoulder-width apart and your arms by your side. Swing both arms forward and then backward. Repeat five times.

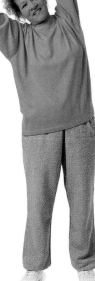

2 Body stretches. Stand with your feet shoulder-width apart. Raise both hands over your head and lean gently to your right, still facing front. Repeat, leaning gently to the left. Stretch five times on each side.

3 Back swings. Stand with your feet shoulder-width apart and clasp your hands in front of your chest with elbows bent and arms level. Slowly rotate your upper body to the left five times, and then repeat to the right. Keep your hips stationary during the exercise.

The PE Teacher

A good physical education (PE) teacher motivates children to take an interest in sports and fitness, giving them the right start for a healthy lifestyle. Understanding educational approaches may help you to encourage your own children to be more active.

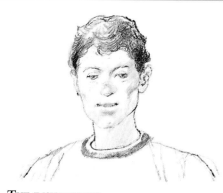

THE INSTRUCTOR
Over the last decade the incidence of child obesity has increased dramatically, and the decline of team sports and physical education has to some extent been blamed. Today's PE teacher has the difficult task of motivating children to take an interest in sports when, due to today's more sedentary lifestyles, they may be lacking in fitness and enthusiasm.

SHOWING THE WAY
A PE teacher is responsible for ensuring that children know how to exercise safely without damaging growing muscles. A guided warm-up at the start of the class and cooling down at the end are essential.

Educators today recognize the importance of establishing healthy lifestyles for children, but they are also aware of the vital role of motivation. Much of the current thinking behind physical education programs focuses on getting every child directly involved. Small group games are often promoted rather than activities that involve a whole class, so that no child misses out on participating. Even if a child is unable to take an active part in a lesson, he or she is still encouraged to attend the play session and help plan activities or evaluate other children's work.

What qualifications do you need to become a physical education teacher?
Entrance into PE teaching is possible through a number of routes, but you generally need at least an undergraduate degree. It could be a Bachelor of Arts in Education with a major focus of study in physical education, or it could be within another discipline followed by postgraduate work to obtain a certificate for teaching. Students of physical education learn about health and physiology, human movement, education, and teaching practices. It is also possible to take the degree with PE options at both the primary and secondary levels.

What sort of clothing should children wear?
Many schools have a PE uniform of shorts and short-sleeve tops; Sneakers are important footwear, and track suits are encouraged for outdoor games and athletics, particularly during cold winter months. Children should not wear jewelery while playing, as this can increase the chance of injury.

What activities are children taught at school?
Children are taught at various degrees of complexity and intensity throughout their primary and secondary years, starting off at the simplest levels of participation and understanding and gradually building up to more advanced levels of individual and team competition. While physical education curricu-

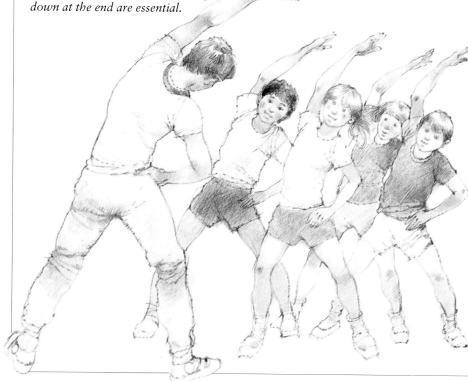

lums vary according to the resources available in a community, most are structured around activities aimed at providing a broad range of exercise experience. The following may be included: games, gymnastics, dance, athletic activities, swimming, and general or adventure outdoor activities. All of these aim to build children's fitness levels and motor, or movement, skills, but some areas have specific additional areas of focus. Games, for example, aim to develop co-operation and effective communication with others, as well as concepts of fair play and the application of rules. Gymnastics, on the other hand, are specifically directed at developing controlled body movement, strength, and flexibility. Dance tries to help children learn about movement as a medium for expression, while athletics focuses on particular motor skills such as running, jumping, and throwing. Swimming develops breathing techniques and particular muscle groups. Outdoor adventure activities give children a chance to face challenges in a natural environment, building confidence and initiative. Adventure activities are also particularly good for increasing enthusiasm and motivation.

All of these areas of activity are designed to increase children's awareness of the general themes of health and fitness, meeting personal and group challenges, and developing a positive attitude to physical activity.

How does a teacher develop interesting activities for children of different age groups?

Teachers structure activities to match the psychological and physical stage of development of their children. For example, in a games class for seven-year-olds the children might be taught how to develop their skills in throwing and catching and playing easy games. Complicated rules and skills can be too difficult for younger children to understand and could result in the loss of their interest.

At age 10 children are introduced to particular skills such as controlling a ball while moving, and to new concepts such as marking an opponent. By 9 or 10 years of age, most children are taking part in team sports, such as football, baseball, hockey, and soccer, and are expected to understand the basic principles. Children ages 11 and up are usually encouraged to keep building their skills in various sports and to try out for teams that compete with those of other schools.

In dance classes, nine-year-olds are taught about contrasting movements, for example traveling, turning, or making arm gestures; at age 10 they may start to learn about moving in set patterns, following one movement with another; and by the age of 12 they are usually learning how to move and shape the body to suggest a certain character or an emotion.

How do teachers motivate reluctant children?

Teachers use a lot of patience to encourage reluctant or embarrassed children to take part in activities, while at the same time not ignoring the needs of the rest of the class. Children who feel self-conscious or inadequate may be put into easy situations within teams of children who have mixed abilities, so they will not feel useless or unwanted. They can help develop rules for a game, for example, or adapt existing rules to make a game fairer. By giving children tasks at which they can succeed, their confidence is boosted and a positive attitude is fostered. Teachers usually try to develop an atmosphere of support during lessons so that children of every level can enjoy themselves without fear of negative criticism or undue pressure.

WHAT YOU CAN DO AT HOME

Try to build on your child's enthusiasm for a particular school sport. If he or she is on a team, expect attendance at all practice sessions and games, and try to be there yourself when parents are invited to watch competitions. You could also investigate community clubs in your area that your child could join after school. Many clubs offer coaching and skills development to improve a child's proficiency. It might also be helpful to look at ways in which the whole family can share an activity so that everyone exercises together—which is good for your activity level as well as theirs. If your child enjoys dancing, for example, investigate the possibility of local dance nights that the family could attend. Getting the whole family involved will reinforce what your children are learning at school, and show your support and pride in what they are achieving. This can help to increase their confidence, which in turn will improve their ability and enjoyment.

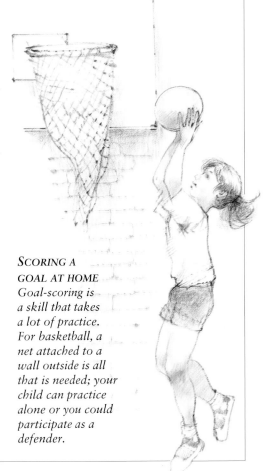

*SCORING A GOAL AT HOME
Goal-scoring is a skill that takes a lot of practice. For basketball, a net attached to a wall outside is all that is needed; your child can practice alone or you could participate as a defender.*

DIET AND THE ELDERLY

Elderly people have conflicting dietary needs. On the one hand they need fewer calories and less volume of food than they did in their younger days, but on the other hand they require just as many nutrients. The food they eat, therefore, must be nutrient dense to provide all the necessary elements—especially minerals, vitamins, and fiber.

Some older people may have neither the budget nor inclination to cook elaborate dishes with costly ingredients. Roast beef with all the usual trimmings may be fine for entertaining but is hardly practical for day-to-day cooking.

Soups can provide convenience, nutrient density, and low price. A blender or food processor is all that is needed to turn everyday ingredients, including leftovers, into a filling, healthful dish. Homemade soups have a distinct advantage over canned ones. Using fresh, unprocessed ingredients allows you to control levels of salt and sugar and preserve nutrients that are often lost in processing. Try pea soup, made with frozen peas, onion, lettuce, mint, and water, with some plain yogurt stirred in at the last minute if you like. You could also substitute vegetables like broccoli or carrots for the peas.

scious children), joining another type of club can still be beneficial. Drama or art may not promote fitness to the same extent as sports, but research shows that almost any activity burns more calories than watching television. Children will also be less tempted to eat while taking part in an activity outside the home than while sitting in front of a television set.

When trying to improve children's diet and exercise habits it is important to avoid criticism and to offer support and encouragement at all times. Youngsters need to feel that good dietary habits and exercise are enjoyable and positive rather than associated with negative feelings. It is also possible to make a child obsessive about weight. Today, children as young as six and seven are placing themselves on diets. Balance and proportion are the keys, and gradual rather than dramatic changes provide the best long-term results.

AVOIDING WEIGHT GAIN THROUGHOUT LIFE

Many people gain weight as they age, but recent research has shown this needn't be inevitable. While the body's metabolic rate does slow down after the mid to late 30s, the main reason that people gain weight seems to be a reduction in exercise and general levels of activity.

For women, menopause also leads to changes in fat distribution, due to a drop in the level of estrogen (see page 19). At this time of life, fat begins to collect around the waist and on the abdomen.

By understanding that the body now needs fewer calories, you can make changes at this crucial time and prevent or at least reduce weight gain. Stopping weight gain before it happens will involve far less effort than trying to lose weight later on.

Stay as active as possible as you grow older. Exercise is still a major factor in a healthy life, helping to increase joint mobility and alleviate the symptoms of arthritis. In fact, you should be more active during middle age to burn off the extra calories that your slower metabolism is not using.

You should also make dietary changes—cut down on high-calorie foods, especially those high in fat and sugar that offer little nutritional value, and increase your level of complex carbohydrates. As you grow older, you may find it hard to digest three main meals and prefer to take a smaller and oftener approach.

Knowing your needs

Identifying your specific nutritional needs and adapting your food intake accordingly is a lifelong commitment. If for example, you become ill and are bedridden, the nutritional value of your food needs to be high but your calorie intake should be reduced because you are completely inactive. If you find it difficult to include exercise or other activity in your day, a similar adjustment should be made. Conversely, it is important to maintain a healthy weight and not let it fall too low, as evidence suggests that fractures associated with osteoporosis are more likely among thin women.

EXERCISE AND AGE
Regular exercise is very important for the elderly. It can prevent the weight gain that often accompanies a slower pace of life after retirement and help keep bones strong and joints supple.

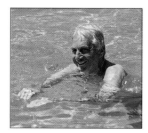

CHAPTER 4

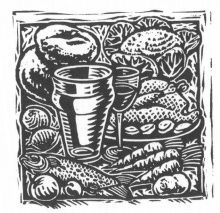

FOODS AND YOUR WEIGHT

It is hardly surprising that so many people find it hard to lose weight, when the popular image of a diet is obsessive calorie counting and tiny portions of unappealing foods. By changing the balance of the types of food you eat you can lose weight—or gain it if you need to—and still enjoy your meals without having to weigh every mouthful.

Food types and your weight

For successful weight control, it helps to be aware of the varying effects that the different food components—carbohydrates, proteins, fiber, and fats—have on your appetite and weight.

When planning meals for a weight-loss regimen, there are two essential ingredients for success: One is that the foods you choose must be relatively low in calories while delivering a high level of nutrients. The other is that meals should be tasty, enjoyable, and satisfying so they don't leave you feeling hungry. Otherwise it will be difficult to stay with the plan for an extended period, and the temptation to revert to old habits may be very strong.

FILLING UP

Many people can successfully introduce healthy, low-fat main dishes into their diets, but find that they still crave dessert, even when their stomachs are full. This is because the part of the brain that controls appetite may register satisfaction from one type of food but still signal some remaining appetite if a different type is available. For this reason, a glimpse of the pastry trolley or the waitress asking if anyone would like dessert is often enough to persuade you that you are still hungry.

Another reason you may still feel like dessert after eating a perfectly satisfying main course is that it takes time for food to digest and be converted to energy in the body. If you wait about half an hour after a main course you will usually feel less like eating anything else. Similarly, you will also be less likely to want second helpings if you wait for a while after the first serving.

The role of fiber

Many studies have shown that foods low in calories for their weight and high in fiber and water, such as apples and baked potatoes, fill people up more quickly than those that are high in calories for their weight and low in fiber and water—croissants, for example. Because it provides a feeling of fullness, fiber is an important component of any weight-loss diet. However, the satisfied feeling does wear off quickly as fiber passes through the system, so each meal should contain modest amounts of protein and fat, which take longer to digest. Hunger will not then return so soon afterward.

Fiber, which is the indigestible part of edible plants, stays in the colon after fat carbohydrate, and protein have been digested,

DIETARY PROPORTIONS

Eating a balanced diet means eating the right proportions of each food type. The illustrated section of this chart shows the percentage of carbohydrates, protein, and fats that should make up your daily diet. The outer, plain-colored section shows, on average, what most people actually do eat.

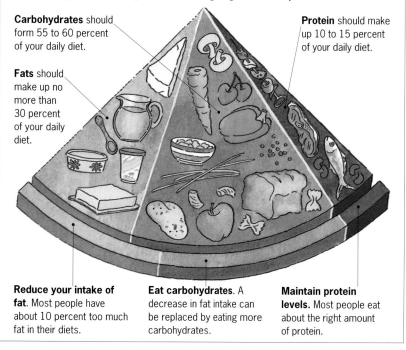

Carbohydrates should form 55 to 60 percent of your daily diet.

Fats should make up no more than 30 percent of your daily diet.

Protein should make up 10 to 15 percent of your daily diet.

Reduce your intake of fat. Most people have about 10 percent too much fat in their diets.

Eat carbohydrates. A decrease in fat intake can be replaced by eating more carbohydrates.

Maintain protein levels. Most people eat about the right amount of protein.

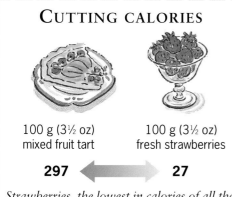

CUTTING CALORIES

100 g (3½ oz)
mixed fruit tart

100 g (3½ oz)
fresh strawberries

297 ⬅➡ **27**

Strawberries, the lowest in calories of all the berries, can still satisfy a sweet tooth.

where it increases the fluid content of stools and prevents constipation. It plays other roles in good health, too, such as helping protect against colon cancer and lowering cholesterol levels (see page 51).

Although there are no established dietary guidelines for fiber, the National Cancer Institute recommends consuming 20 to 35 grams per day. The best way to obtain an adequate amount is to eat at least five to eight servings of fruits and vegetables each day, preferably with their skins, and select whole-grain cereals and breads over those that are highly processed. Nuts and edible seeds such as pumpkin, sesame, and sunflower are also good sources of fiber, though they are relatively high in fat also.

When adding more fiber to your diet, it is important to do it gradually and spread it throughout the day. A sudden increase or consuming too much all at once can result in gasiness, bloating, or abdominal cramps. In some people, particularly the elderly, it can even lead to bowel obstruction.

Too much bran and other insoluble fibers can prevent the digestive system from absorbing certain minerals properly, particularly calcium, iron, and zinc. This is rarely a problem and is unlikely to occur unless more than 35g of fiber a day are consumed.

PROTEINS AND YOUR WEIGHT

Protein, the major structural material of the body, is vital for the maintenance of cells, tissues, and organs, for muscle strength, and the health of hair, skin, and nails. It is also a major component of the enzymes and hormones that regulate the body's metabolism.

When protein is digested, it is broken down into its constituent building blocks known as amino acids. These are transported around the body to be used as needed. The remainder of the protein molecule is essentially sugar, and this is used either for energy—it provides 4 calories per gram, the same as carbohydrates—or stored as glycogen in the liver and muscles.

The needs for protein differ according to the individual. For example, protein requirements are higher for children, athletes, and

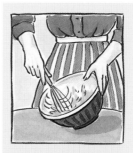

QUICK FITNESS TIP
Instead of using labor-saving devices like food processors and electric mixers, burn some calories by chopping, blending, and whisking by hand.

NEGATIVE CALORIE FOODS

No food contains negative calories—that is, burns more calories in being digested than it actually provides itself. However, some foods such as celery contain so few calories that you can eat as much as you like without putting your weight-control program at risk.

Most fruits and vegetables are relatively low in calories (see page 67), so they are an important part of any weight-control regimen. Packed with vitamins and minerals, they make healthy snacks that can help you to stave off hunger pangs. By filling up on vegetables you will be more able to resist the temptation to eat sugary, high-fat snacks, which are loaded with calories and yet offer little or no nutritional value.

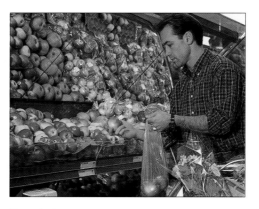

PICK 'N' MIX
Try a variety of fruits and vegetables. Many supermarkets now stock exotic types like chipotle squash or casaba melon as well as familiar favorites. Keep a supply of vegetables in the freezer, too, so you don't run short.

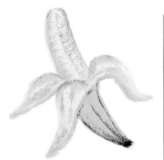

CHOOSE A BANANA
Bananas are a healthy choice if you crave something sweet. Although they are higher in calories than some other fruits, they are a rich source of potassium, which helps maintain normal blood pressure and regulate the body's balance of fluids, and is also essential for many metabolic processes.

people suffering from illness or disease. Protein intake should also be increased during pregnancy and breast feeding. It's recommended that protein make up between 10 and 15 percent of total calories daily.

High-protein foods include meat, poultry, fish, eggs, and dairy foods. If you are eating sufficient protein there is no evidence that eating more will build up muscle without added exercise. Instead, the extra protein will be used to provide energy, and the fat you eat, rather than being used for energy, will be stored. Also, too much protein accelerates calcium excretion.

CARBOHYDRATES AND WEIGHT
The main function of carbohydrates is to provide energy for the body—one gram produces four calories. Many important vitamins and minerals are also found in high-carbohydrate foods. Current dietary recommendations suggest that between 55 and 60 per cent of daily calorie intake should be consumed as carbohydrates, preferably the complex carbohydrates found in potatoes, rice, pasta, cereals, and breads. However, the accompaniments must be relatively low in fat. People who load on the butter, sour cream, or a rich, high-fat sauce, are beefing up the calories. At the same time, the simple carbohydrates prevalent in cookies and candy should be reduced to no more than 10 percent of calories. These provide a quick burst of energy, but then blood

sugar drops quickly back to its previous level and hunger returns in a short time.

After carbohydrates have been digested, they are broken down into simple sugars, and any extras are stored as glycogen in the liver or muscle. Although it is metabolically possible to convert carbohydrate to fat, this rarely occurs.

Diets very low in carbohydrates can be dangerous, possibly leading to mineral imbalances, hypoglycemia, and interference with the efficiency of the body's metabolism. Some people who have tried low-carbohydrate diets have reported experiencing dizzy spells, nausea, fatigue, and depression.

FATS AND YOUR WEIGHT
Fats store extra energy in the body, aid in absorbing the fat soluble vitamins A,D, E, and K, help maintain cell membranes, are used in the production of certain hormones, insulate the body against cold, and protect vital organs. They are made up of three types of fatty acids—saturated, monunsaturated, and polyunsaturated. Although all fats are a combination of these three, one type usually predominates. Most animal fats are mainly saturated and most vegetable fats are primarily unsaturated.

The amount of fat we actually need is miniscule—about 1 tablespoon per day of polyunsaturated fat that contains the essential fatty acids, or EFA, linolenic acid and linoleic acid. (The EFAs are plentiful in seeds, nuts, and most vegetable oils except olive oil.) If we limited our intake to such a small amount of fat, most of our food would be dry and tasteless and our meals less satisfying. However, many persons eat far more than is healthful. Fat should comprise no more than 30 percent of daily intake, with a maximum of 10 percent of this amount coming from saturated fats. In a daily caloric intake of about 2,000 calories, this would be about 60 grams of total fat and about 20 grams of saturated fat.

Saturated fats, found in meat, whole-milk dairy products, and coconut and palm oils, are implicated in raising cholesterol levels in the body, whereas monounsaturated fats, found in nuts and olive oil, help to lower cholesterol levels. Another fat, transfatty acid, is a by product of hydrogenation and is found in some margarines and shortening. Transfatty acids have been linked both to coronary heart disease and cancer.

This competitive but social game can be played with one partner (singles) or in a group of four (doubles). It improves lower body strength and endurance while demanding muscle coordination.

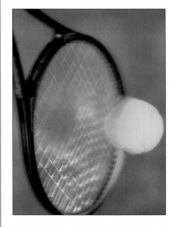

MUSCLE GROUPS BENEFITING
The lower torso and legs benefit the most. The upper torso, shoulders, and arms are stretched during strokes.

EQUIPMENT
Shorts and T-shirt. Well-fitted and supportive tennis shoes are advisable.

CALORIES BURNT
Singles: about 7 calories per minute, (420 per hour). Doubles: about 6 calories per minute (360 per hour).

PLANNING YOUR MEALS TO GAIN WEIGHT

If you are 15 percent or more below your ideal weight range and feel unduly fatigued and frequently chilly or, if you are a woman and have missed three or more consecutive periods, you ought to consult your doctor about the possible need to gain weight. A diet for safely gaining should follow basic healthy eating principles, with 50 to 65 percent of calories coming from carbohydrates and more modest amounts from fat and protein. A dramatic weight gain should be avoided, just as dramatic weight loss should be. The aim should be a gradual, steady increase. A sensible calorie intake would be about 3,000 calories per day. These can be divided into three main meals and two or three snacks.

Increasing and maintaining weight levels is difficult without regular physical exercise. Muscles are more dense than fat, so muscle-building exercise is the best for weight gain. Appetite may diminish at the start of training but will increase again after a few days.

SAMPLE DAILY MENU FOR WEIGHT GAIN
The menu shown here provides a day's balanced diet, following healthy eating rules and supplying a total intake of 3,196 calories. It includes several rich sources of protein and carbohydrates, but is not too high in fat.

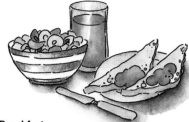

Breakfast
50 g (1¾ oz) cornflakes with dried fruit topping and 200 ml (6.8 fl oz) low-fat (2%) milk; two slices of toast with jam and 2 tsp polyunsaturated margarine; 200 ml (6.8 fl oz) fresh orange juice = 736 calories

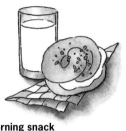

Mid morning snack
Bagel with 25 g (1oz) cream cheese, and 225 ml (8 fl oz) low-fat (2%) milk = 392 calories

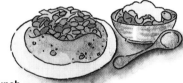

Lunch
Baked potato with 250 g (9 oz) baked beans and grated Cheddar cheese topping; 125 g (4½ oz) fruit salad with 125 g (4½ oz) custard made with low-fat (2%) milk = 790 calories

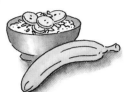

Afternoon snack
125 g (4½ oz) bowl of low-fat rice pudding and one sliced banana = 214 calories

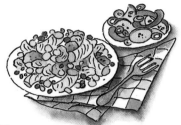

Dinner
Seafood pasta with 250 g (8¾ oz) boiled pasta, 90 g (3¼ oz) canned tuna in water, 85 g (3 oz) peas, 90 g (3¼ oz) sweetcorn, 200 g (7 oz) canned tomatoes, mixed herbs; salad with lettuce, tomatoes, cucumber, green onions, watercress, red and green peppers, olive oil and balsamic vinegar dressing = 682 calories

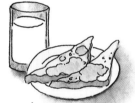

Evening snack
Two slices of toast with 30 g (1⅛ oz) peanut butter and 225 ml (8 fl oz) low-fat (2%) milk = 382 calories

---

Any fat that you eat above your basic energy requirements will be stored on your body as fat. The only way to get rid of it is to decrease the calories that you eat and increase the calories that you burn by doing more exercise. Develop a habit of checking the labels on food packaging to determine what kind of fats and how many are contained in the food. When a label claims that a food is fat-free, it must by law contain no more than ½ gram of fat per serving.

New synthetic fats are being developed that have fewer calories than natural fats, which provide nine calories per gram, or more than twice as much as protein or carbohydrate. The best known is Olestra (see page 74), which is now used in some snacks such as potato chips in the United States.

VITAMINS AND MINERALS AND WEIGHT

Whether you are trying to lose or gain weight, amidst concerns about counting calories it is easy to forget about the vitamins and minerals that are essential to maintain good health. Especially when you eat less food, you need to select carefully to ensure that the ones you choose have a high nutrient density. If you are in any doubt, consult a doctor or dietitian for advice. A multivitamin and/or mineral supplement may be recommended.

A healthy body is easier to maintain at a desirable weight because bodily functions are more efficient. Therefore, getting your essential nutrients can be a big help in your weight-control program.

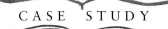
The Empty Calorie Eater

Many people who are overweight may not eat more food than people who are slim, but they eat the wrong types—foods that are high in fat and sugar and low in fiber. This type of eating, known as an empty calorie diet, contains relatively few whole-grain cereals, fruits, and vegetables and therefore provides a lot of energy but very few essential vitamins and minerals.

Ted is a 66-year-old man who, since retiring, has put on an excessive number of pounds and is now unhealthily overweight. He has always been a little on the plump side, but was managing to keep his weight within reasonable limits by walking to work every day and participating in a varied social life with his workmates. However, now that he finds himself with a less structured day, he lounges about the house most of the time—watching television, reading the newspaper, and snacking frequently. The combination of very little physical activity, other than walking down the road to the local shops, and excess weight is making him less mobile, and he is starting to find that he is short of breath much of the time. Ted is also eating all the wrong kinds of food. Apart from a reasonably balanced evening meal, he consumes foods that are high in calories and fat and low in essential vitamins, minerals, and fiber. He generally has a very light breakfast, but then fills up on cookies or crackers until lunchtime, when he has a meal that includes fried bacon or sausages. He rarely eats any vegetables before dinner other than deep-fried chips. Ted also drinks about four cans of beer a day. His wife, Sheila, who would also like to lose weight, has suggested that Ted make an appointment with their doctor. After an initial consultation, Ted's doctor referred him to a registered dietitian for a more thorough dietary assessment. Ted was asked to record his food intake for one week, so that the dietitian could analyze the results for calories and fat, protein, carbohydrate, and alcohol content. After careful examination, the dietitian advised Ted to alter his diet and increase his level of physical activity by doing more frequent exercise.

LIFESTYLE
Having an unstructured day can lead to weight gain. People can easily become sedentary, which slows down their metabolic rate so that even fewer calories are burned and more are laid down as fat.

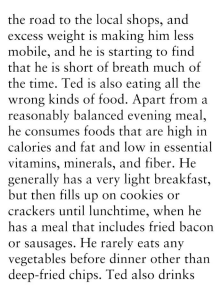

FOOD
Eating the wrong kinds of food will not only add unnecessary weight but will also contribute to other health problems such as high cholesterol.

PARTNER/SPOUSE
It is much easier to lose weight if a close family member agrees to lose weight too.

EXERCISE
Being overweight can limit your physical abilities. This is a problem after retirement, when you may wish to take up new activities.

RETIREMENT
Eating more and doing less exercise is a common cause of weight gain after stopping work.

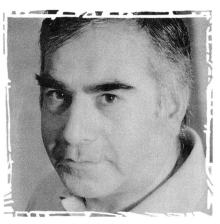

WHAT SHOULD TED DO?

Ted needs to cut down on fats and sugars and increase complex carbohydrates, fruits, and vegetables in his diet. He should replace his usual breakfast of white toast and butter with whole-wheat cereal or porridge, accompanied by low-fat or skim milk and very little sugar . This will fill him up more. He should also use low-fat milk in his tea and coffee.

For lunches Ted should replace the fried foods with salads, lean meat or fish, and low-fat dairy products. When he craves snacks or a dessert he should eat fruit, sorbet, or low-fat yogurt and not his usual cookies, chocolate bar, or cake, but allow himself a treat now and then. For his main meals Ted should eat plenty of vegetables, with pasta, rice, or potatoes (not fried) for carbohydrates, and beans, chicken, fish, or lean meat for protein.

Any weight-loss plan must aim to reduce alcohol intake and Ted should definitely attempt to cut his beer drinking to one can per day. He should also try to cut down on the hours he spends watching television, as this is when he tends to snack. He could replace some of his television time with regular exercise, for instance, a daily 30- to 60-minute walk. Gardening would be another way of getting more activity into his life.

Action Plan

PARTNER/SPOUSE
Discuss weight loss plans with Sheila, because she also wants to lose weight. Work out shopping lists and prepare meals together.

RETIREMENT
Plan ways of making better use of free time on a daily basis, including more physical activity. Take up a new hobby or do volunteer work in the community.

FOOD
Change diet to reduce fatty and sugary foods. Eat more fruits, vegetables, and complex carbohydrates. Experiment with new recipes.

LIFESTYLE
Make a list of achievable goals toward a healthier lifestyle that can be attained over the next few months, such as gradually cutting down on the hours spent watching television and using more time for active pursuits.

EXERCISE
Start an exercise program. Choose enjoyable activities and try to exercise daily for at least 30 minutes.

HOW THINGS TURNED OUT FOR TED

Ted, with the help of his wife Sheila, changed his diet along the lines recommended by the dietitian. In time, both he and Sheila came to enjoy their new way of eating and looked forward to preparing new and exciting meals together each evening.

As part of their healthier lifestyle, they made a point of walking every morning for 30 minutes to an hour in the local park. On the weekends they started going for longer, more varied walks out in the countryside, even joining a local hiking club.

Within six months, Ted had lost 10 kg (22 lb) and Sheila had also lost weight. His mobility gradually improved with the regular exercise and he became less breathless. This meant that he was able to walk at a quicker pace and he began to enjoy his morning walks more than before. The pair are now very keen walkers and have taken a number of short holidays based around interesting walks. This gives them something to plan for and look forward to, providing physical and mental exercise.

Ted has more energy today and is able to do the things he had planned for his retirement, such as redecorating the house, helping out at a local boys' club, and growing many of the vegetables that now form a large part of his and Sheila's diet.

FOODS AND THEIR CALORIC VALUES

In order to keep the fat content of your diet to 30 percent or less per day, you need to know about how much fat is contained in each food you eat. Studies have shown that most people are poor judges of calorie and fat content. This chart can help you make better judgments about these two factors. To calculate fat percentage, multiply fat grams by nine, then divide this figure by the number of calories. For example, if Brie has 8 grams of fat, 8 x 9 = 72 ÷ 100 = 72 percent fat.

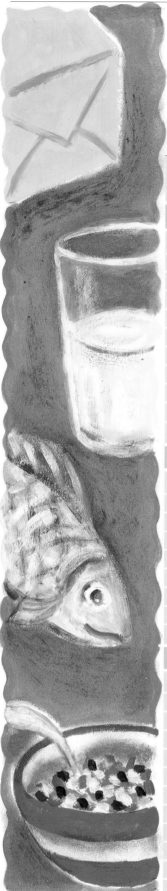

FOOD GROUP	CALORIES per 100 g (3½ oz)	FAT g per 100 g (3½ oz)	AVERAGE SERVING SIZE	CALORIES (per serving)	FAT (g per serving)
DAIRY PRODUCTS					
Brie, double cream	400	32	25 g/1 oz	100	8.0
Butter	728	82	1 tbsp, 14 g/½ oz	102	11.5
Cheese, Cheddar	412	34.4	50 g/1¾ oz	206	17.2
Cheese, cottage	98	3.9	50 g/1¾ oz	49	2
Cheese, cream, low-fat	200	17	25 g/1 oz	60	5.0
Cheese, Edam	333	25.4	50 g/1¾ oz	166	12.7
Margarine	728	82	1 tbsp, 14 g/½ oz	102	11.5
Milk, skim	33	0.1	1 glass, 200 ml/7 fl oz	66	0.2
Milk, whole	66	3.9	1 glass, 200 ml/7 fl oz	132	7.8
Yogurt, with fruit	90	0.7	150 g/5¼ oz	135	1.1
Yogurt, plain, low-fat	52	1	150 g/5¼ oz	78	1.5
MEAT, FISH, AND LEGUMES					
Beef, roasted rib	214	12	100 g/3½ oz	214	12
Chicken, roasted	216	14	115 g/4 oz	248	16.1
Lamb, roasted	266	17.9	100 g/3½ oz	266	17.9
Lentils, red	100	0.4	100 g/3½ oz	100	0.4
Pork sausages, grilled	318	24.6	100 g/3½ oz	318	24.6
Cod, baked	96	1.2	150 g/5¼ oz	144	1.8
Mackerel, broiled	188	10.5	150 g/5¼ oz	324	15.75
Salmon, poached	197	4.6	150 g/5¼ oz	296	6.9
Tuna, in water	122	1.6	150 g/5¼ oz	210	4.0
CEREAL PRODUCTS					
Rice, boiled brown	110	1.0	130 g/4½ oz	144	1.3
Bran flakes	303	1.7	35 g/1¼ oz	106	0.6
Bread, whole wheat	215	2.5	2 slices, 70 g/2½ oz	151	1.75
Bread, white	235	1.9	2 slices, 70 g/2½ oz	165	1.33
Cereal, muesli	363	5.9	40 g/1½ oz	145	2.4
Cereal, puffed rice	369	0.9	40 g/1½ oz	148	0.4
Crackers, saltine	400	15	30 g/1⅛ oz	120	3.0
Crackers, whole-wheat	466	16.6	30 g/1⅛	140	5.0
Pizza, cheese and tomato	277	8.3	2 slices, 130 g/4½ oz	306	10.8
Popcorn, air popped	483	5.0	12 g/½ oz	58	0.6
Spaghetti, marinara	104	0.7	150 g/5¼ oz	156	1.1
Tofu, steamed	73	4.2	100 g/3½ oz	73	4.2

FOOD GROUP	CALORIES per 100 g	FAT g per 100 g	AVERAGE SERVING SIZE	CALORIES (per serving)	FAT (g per serving)
FRUITS AND VEGETABLES					
Apple, 1 medium	62	0.1	130 g/4½ oz	80	0.6
Banana, 1 medium	95	0.3	130 g/4½ oz	124	0.39
Nectarine, 1 medium	40	0.1	130 g/4½ oz	52	0.1
Orange, 1 medium	37	0.1	100 g/3½ oz	37	0.1
Peach, 1 medium	33	0.1	140 g/5 oz	46	0.1
Beans, baked	84	0.6	100 g/3½ oz	84	0.6
Broccoli, steamed	29	0.7	150 g/5¼ oz	44	1.0
Carrots, boiled	24	0.4	100 g/3½ oz	24	0.4
Celery, raw	7	0.2	50 g/1¾ oz	3.5	0.1
Cucumbers	10	0.1	50 g/1¾ oz	5	0.05
Green peppers, raw	15	0.3	50 g/1¾ oz	7.5	0.15
Lettuce	14	0.5	50 g/1¾ oz	7	0.25
Mushrooms, raw	29	Nil	50 g/1¾ oz	14	Nil
Potato, large, baked	110	0.1	200 g/7 oz	220	0.2
Potato, medium, boiled	69	Negligible	150 g/5¼ oz	104	0.1
Potatoes, french fried	239	12.4	150 g/5¼ oz	359	18.6
Potatoes, mashed	104	4.3	150 g/5¼ oz	156	6.5
Tomatoes, 2 medium	31	0.3	70 g/2½ oz	22	0.2
DRINKS					
Beer, regular	32	Negligible	1 can, 355/12 fl oz	150	Negligible
Bloody Mary	46	0.13	1 glass, 150 ml/5 fl oz	116	0.2
Cola	39	Nil	1 can, 355 ml/12 fl oz	129	Nil
Gin and tonic	80	Nil	1 glass, 220 ml/7½ fl oz	171	Nil
Ginger ale	33	Nil	1 can, 355 ml/12 fl oz	113	Nil
Lemonade	47	Nil	1 glass, 230 ml/8 fl oz	107	Nil
Martini	218	Nil	75 ml/2½ fl oz	274	Nil
Wine, red	68	Nil	1 glass, 125 ml/4 fl oz	85	Nil
Wine, white, dry	66	Nil	1 glass, 125 ml/4 fl oz	82	Nil
Wine, white, sweet	94	Nil	1 glass, 125 ml/4 fl oz	117	Nil
SNACKS					
Chocolate bar	529	30.3	25 g/1 oz	132	7.6
Potato chips	546	37.6	30 g/1⅛ oz	164	11.3
Crackers, cheese	500	26.6	30 g/1⅛ oz	150	8
Low fat potato chips	483	21.5	30 g/1⅛ oz	145	6.5
Peanuts, roasted in oil	602	53	40 g/1½ oz	241	21.2
CONDIMENTS					
Mayonnaise	707	78.5	1 tbsp/14 g	99	11
Mustard, brown	100	3.0	1 tsp/5 g	5	0.3
Olive oil	707	78.5	1 tbsp/14 g	99	11
Salad dressing, French	412	38.7	1 tbsp/14 g	66	6.2
Tomato ketchup	98	Negligible	1 tbsp/14 g	15	Negligible

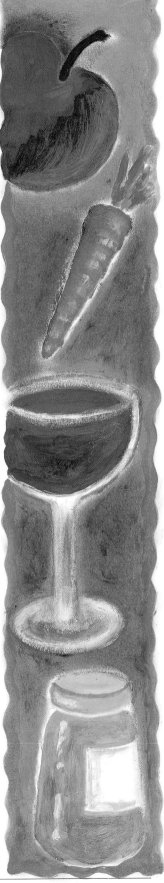

The Obesity Dietitian

Dietitians provide nutritional advice to people with a range of ailments for whom changes in diet can help to improve their health. Some dietitians—often called obesity dietitians—specialize in helping people whose weight is a health problem in itself.

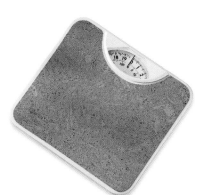

WEIGHTY MATTERS
Scales are an important part of a dietitian's armory—essential for charting a patient's overall progress—but they should not be over-relied upon. To be healthy, weight loss should be gradual. Lifestyle changes are more important than shedding pounds quickly.

Dietitians recognize that there are many different reasons for people being overweight. As therapists, they try to treat patients as individuals, encouraging them to discuss the problem before listening to advice. Besides making dietary recommendations, dietitians may also spend some time talking about positive lifestyle changes that can help a person achieve an acceptable weight and maintain it at that level.

HELPING THE DIETITIAN
It will help the dietitian to have a detailed breakdown of exactly what you eat. To make sure you remember everything, keep a diary of all the food and beverages you consume for a few weeks. This can then be used in your first consultation.

What sort of training do obesity dietitians have?
In the U.S. dietitians who specialize in weight loss are usually registered dietitians and members of the American Dietetic Association. They have a degree with a specialty in dietetics and have completed a 900-hour supervised internship. Their training covers treatment of obesity in depth, and usually they must attend additional training sessions sponsored by hospitals, nutritional organizations, and research facilities.

What questions might a dietitian ask on the first visit?
Patients who are referred to a dietitian because they wish to lose weight often have other health problems as well. The dietitian will want to know the person's medical history, previous experience with weight-reducing diets, and whether there is a history of obesity in the family. He or she will then assess current food intake and eating patterns. For example, does the patient normally have breakfast, and are mealtimes regular or sporadic? Finally, the dietitian may want to discuss in detail why the patient wishes to lose weight. This might seem like an unnecessary question, but it can help establish the strength of a patient's motivation.

What dietary advice is given to overweight patients?
Dietary advice is carefully tailored to an individual's needs, so it can vary tremendously, depending upon the

patient's current food intake, lifestyle, the amount of weight that has to be lost, and whether there is any other medical condition to take into account. Generally speaking, however, patients are encouraged to make gradual changes to their diet, incorporating more vegetables, fruits, and whole-grain cereals and reducing the proportion of foods that contain a lot of fat and sugar. Most dietitians do not ask people to count calories but encourage them instead to concentrate on making healthier food choices, which they and their family can enjoy. In this way the diet gradually becomes part of the patient's usual lifestyle.

Where do dietitians see their patients?

Dietitians work in private practice, hospital out-patient clinics, and community centers. Patients may be seen either as individuals or in groups. For example, a dietitian may give talks to groups of patients attending a coronary rehabilitation class, or at education sessions organized for patients with diabetes. Dietitians who see patients in private practice, usually do so on an individual basis, which allows them to give more one-to-one attention.

How many appointments do patients usually have?

This depends on the nature of the problem. Some patients may be seen regularly, once a week or fortnight for an indefinite period of time, if the causes of their weight problems are complex and they are benefiting from a lot of support. Alternatively, after the initial assessment and one follow-up appointment, a patient may be referred back to her primary care physician, who will then monitor the person's progress, following the dietitian's advice.

Dietitians spend much of their time training nurses in how to help overweight and obese patients, and these nurses are usually very good at offering long-term support and practical advice.

Are there any special techniques that dietitians use?

Yes, many of them use what are called behavioral therapy techniques to help their patients gain greater control over their eating habits. This is not as complicated as it sounds. It simply involves working out some basic rules to help people eat when they are hungry and not for emotional reasons or from poor habits. For example, if you discuss with a dietitian that you feel a constant urge to snack, you may be advised to restrict your eating to one room in the house, for example, to the kitchen or dining room. You will then be less likely to think about food when you are sitting in the den or the bedroom, since it is not a place where you normally eat. Similarly, you may be told not to eat while you are engaged in any other activity, for instance, watching television. This is because with time, your mind may connect this particular activity with eating.

Eventually, whenever you sit down to watch television you will feel like having something to eat, whether or not you are hungry. A patient who requires further behavioral therapy may be referred to a psychologist for more specialized treatment.

Do dietitians work with other health professionals?

A dietitian will work closely with your primary care physician or family doctor in order to understand fully any other medical problems you may have. Some dietitians also work with psychologists (see above) in the treatment of obesity. For patients who have specific eating disorders, the psychologist may use cognitive or behavioral therapy (see pages 40–41) to examine the cause of the disorder in depth and discuss potential solutions. Other dietitians work with exercise specialists, who can help a patient effectively combine diet and exercise to achieve the best long-term results.

WHAT YOU CAN DO AT HOME

If you have a tendency to be obsessed with food and find yourself eating even when you're not hungry— perhaps when you are anxious, bored, or frustrated—the tips below may help you develop better eating habits and begin to regain control over your weight.

▶ *Don't eat on the move or while watching TV. Always sit down at a table to eat and try to relax.*

▶ *Serve your meal on a medium-sizeP plate, not a large one. This will make the portions look larger.*

▶ *Immediately after serving yourself, wrap up any leftovers and put them in the refrigerator.*

▶ *Include planned healthy snacks in your diet—a piece of fruit, low-fat yogurt, or something left over from dinner.*

TIMING YOUR MEALS
Eat your meals at the same time each day. You will find that your body quickly adjusts to more regular eating habits and you will feel less inclined to eat between meals.

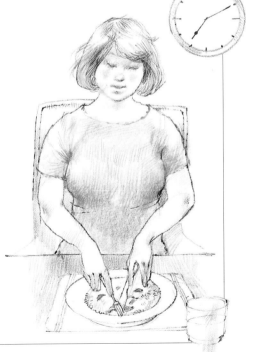

DRINKS AND WEIGHT CONTROL

There are various myths concerning how water, fruit juices, caffeinated drinks, and alcohol can affect weight loss. The truth about which are beneficial to your health is actually very simple.

A high fluid intake is vital for your body to function properly. Water plays a part in nearly all of the body's functions. For this reason it is essential to keep up your fluid intake even when dieting. Some drinks have quite a high calorie content, however, so it is also important to choose low-calorie or calorie-free drinks.

WATER AND DIETING
Many overweight people believe that some of their excess weight is due to water retention and wonder if they should reduce their intake of water or take diuretic pills. The answer to both of these questions is no.

Diuretic pills should be avoided, except under strict medical supervision, as they can lead to dehydration and any weight loss will be temporary. They can also cause the loss of essential nutrients from the body. Whether you are trying to lose weight or not you should aim to drink the equivalent of at least eight glasses of water a day. Some obese people may have an abnormal accumulation of fluid, known as edema, which is indicated by swelling, particularly in the legs, ankles, and feet. The causes of edema are many and can signal a serious underlying condition. Anyone who has edema should consult a doctor as soon as possible.

CALORIE CONTENT OF SOME SOFT DRINKS

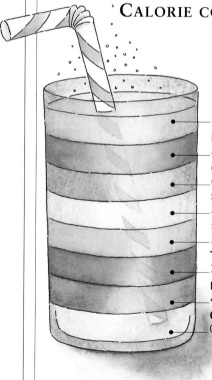

Per 100 ml (3.5 fl oz):

Ginder ale
33 cal, 8.5 g sugar

Fresh orange juice
43 cal, 9.3g sugar

Cranberry juice
65 cal, 16.5 g sugar

Skim milk
38cal, 5.4 g sugar

Sports drink
28 cal, 6.4 g sugar

Tomato juice
14 cal, 3 g sugar

Flavored diet drink
4 cal, no sugar

Carbonated water
0 cal, no sugar

A weight-control plan is not just about the food you consume; beverages can account for a surprising number of calories. What needs to be considered is whether or not they are empty calories. Soft drinks, with or without sugar, contain no nutrients. Fruit juices, though relatively high in sugar, also have some vitamins, especially vitamin C, and small amounts of minerals. There is no doubt that water, which is completely free of calories, is the best drink for a weight watcher. You can drink as much as you like. So, when you are really thirsty, reach for the tap rather than a soft drink.

WHAT'S IN A DRINK?
The calorie and sugar content of beverages vary widely, as is shown in this comparison of eight popular drinks.

CUTTING CALORIES

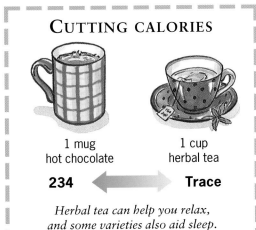

1 mug hot chocolate	1 cup herbal tea
234	**Trace**

Herbal tea can help you relax, and some varieties also aid sleep.

Caffeinated drinks

Caffeine, present in coffee, tea, chocolate, and colas and other soft drinks, stimulates the metabolic rate and can, in theory, help burn calories. However, this effect is generally too small to significantly affect weight loss. Caffeine also stimulates the brain—thus enhancing mental performance—speeds up the heart rate, increases the production of digestive acids, and increases the flow of urine. Because of this last effect, some dieters step up their use of caffeine in the hopes of losing weight by eliminating water from their systems. The loss, of course, is only temporary, and the side effects from too much caffeine can be unpleasant. They include insomnia, jitteriness, and irritability.

Herbal teas provide a healthy alternative, and are virtually calorie free when drunk without milk or sugar.

Alcohol and your weight

Alcohol is high in calories and should be limited as part of a weight-control program. (See page 67 for specific calorie counts of some popular drinks.) One common misconception is that pilsner lagers are lower in calories because more of the sugar is converted to alcohol. However, since 1 g of sugar, containing 4 calories, is converted to 1 g of alcohol, which yields 7 calories, a pilsner lager actually contains more calories than an ordinary lager.

In addition, alcohol can stimulate your appetite. People who are attempting to gain weight are often advised to have an alcoholic drink before a meal. If you are trying to lose weight it is better to avoid alcohol altogether. The influence of alcohol can destroy your willpower and the intention to limit intake to just one or two drinks can quickly disappear. You may also be tempted to eat a high-fat snack which you might otherwise have resisted.

If you are used to drinking alcohol regularly and cannot give it up, allow yourself one drink before or with dinner as part of your whole diet plan, but don't let one drink slip into two or more. See page 53 for tips on how to limit alcohol when on a diet.

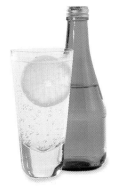

BON APERITIF!
Some people find that drinking carbonated water before a meal partially fills them up and as a result they eat less during the meal.

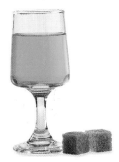

WHICH IS THE LESSER OF TWO EVILS?
When people think about losing weight, they automatically consider cutting back on fat and sugar. Often alcohol is overlooked and some people even congratulate themselves for missing a meal because they were at a bar with colleagues. In fact, alcohol contains almost twice as many calories per gram as sugar, so a liquid supper could cost you your waistline.

FRUIT OR FRUIT JUICE?

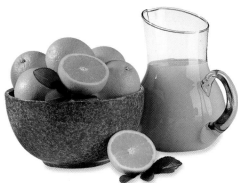

Fruit juices usually contain at least some vitamin C, and therefore are good sources of the vitamin for a person who does not eat many fruits or vegetables. However, for anyone who receives enough vitamin C from whole fruits and vegetables, fruit juice can act simply as a source of calories. It is easy to drink a large amount of juice when you are thirsty, without realizing how many calories you are consuming. Juices are also relatively low in fiber because this is retained in the pulp of the fruit, most of which is discarded during juice extraction. When buying fruit juices, look for unsweetened varieties and try to avoid those that are simply high-sugar soft drinks based on juice concentrate.

WHAT IS THE DIFFERENCE?
1 liter (33.8 fluid oz) of unsweetened orange juice provides about 360 calories, 88 g sugar, 0.4 g fiber, and 390 mg vitamin C. Five large oranges, weighing about the same, when eaten without peel supply 370 calories, 85 g sugar, 17 g fiber, and 540 mg vitamin C.

THE FACTS ABOUT HEALTH FOODS

Are the products in health food stores better for you than those in supermarkets? The answer is—sometimes. Healthful foods are available everywhere; it's important to understand the labels.

Advertising for some health foods implies that their consumption will confer health benefits on the consumer. Many claims are general; others are specifically related to a certain disease or problem. Claims made for health foods can be difficult to substantiate, and their nutritional and caloric values are as variable as those of other foods. The important message is that health foods do not necessarily contain more nutritional value when compared with foods that are not advertised as such. However, used discriminately, they can serve well in a healthful eating plan. The selections in health food stores are usually

above average in nutritional content. You will, for example, find a much greater variety of whole-grain products, fruit juices, low-fat alternatives, organic foods, and nutritional supplements than what is available in even the largest supermarkets. The varied choices can make planning and sticking to a healthful diet easier and more interesting. But you have to read the labels to determine if the fat content is healthful. Labeling laws make it mandatory that all packaged foods state, among other things, just how many fat grams are contained in one serving (see opposite page for how to calculate percentage of fat).

FOOD PACKAGING – BEHIND THE IMAGE

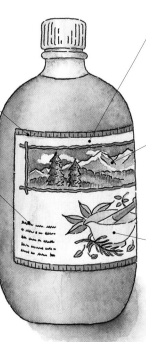

A tape measure, which will catch your eye, is a marketing ploy to make sure you instantly recognize this as a product that can be used as part of a calorie-controlled diet.

Nutritional labels reveal the truth about calorie content and any additives that may not match the healthy image

TRICKS OF THE TRADE
Packaging can be used to convey a healthy image. Words such as "light" and "low-fat" in tall, slim letters will further enhance the message.

Pale colors are used to give the product a clean, almost clinical look. This may be intended to give the impression that it is pure.

Mountain scenery is often pictured to suggest that the product is so natural it has an affinity with nature itself.

Imagery such as a pestle and mortar surrounded by herbs may be used to give the impression that the product is medically good for you.

It is important to be observant when shopping, to ensure that you are not taken in by packaging gimmicks and marketing ploys. There are many approaches that manufacturers use to convince you that their product should be a regular part of your diet. The images presented can be misleading, so you should always read the contents label carefully. Sometimes, when the product is fat-free, more sugar has been used to retain a good taste and texture. With a little experience, you will discover which products are valid for inclusion in your weight-control plan and can really help make your diet healthier.

There is a big caveat concerning nutritional supplements, which are a big part of the stock in health food stores. These products are not regulated by the agency that sets the standards for food labeling, and many of the claims made for supplements have not been substianted by scientific studies.

VALUE OF "NATURAL" FOODS

The term "natural" often appears on food labels. Just exactly what this means is vague. In some cases, the word is used to indicate that there are no chemical additives. In other instances, it may be a synonym for "organic," which means it has met stringent standards to qualify for use of the term. The ingredients in processed foods must be at least 95% organic (except for salt and water) and may not have any artificial ingredients or chemical preservatives like nitrates and sulfates. Such products may be safer because they do not contain any residues of fertilizers and insecticides, but they are not necessarily superior in nutritional content. Also, they spoil more quickly because they lack preservatives.

Another example of a product that is advertised as "natural," but may not offer any greater or lesser health benefits, is bottled water. Tap waters are not pure, but neither are bottled waters, and some contain high levels of minerals that can be unsuitable for children and people with hypertension.

In the same way that labeling of natural foods can be misleading, so can claims for natural or healthy aids to losing weight. Unfortunately, there is no miracle answer in a bottle. (See pages 110–11 for more information concerning dieting aids.)

Low-fat health foods

Many foods bear labels saying reduced fat, low-fat, very low fat, light, or lite. This labeling can be helpful, because the differences between low-fat and regular versions of some products, including yogurt, cheese, and mayonnaise, is often significant. But to find out exactly what the difference is, you must look at the nutritional content on the label, compare it with that of the regular version, and assess for yourself whether it is a worthwhile substitution.

Calculating fat content

To determine if your daily intake of fat is being held to the recommended standard of 30 percent or less each day, you need to know how many grams of fat and how many total calories are present in each serving of food you eat. Packaged foods are required to have this information on their labels. For other food items, you can buy a book that lists these values.

To calculate the percentage of fat in a serving, first find the number of fat grams it contains and multiply that number by 9 (the number of calories in one gram of fat). Then, divide the number of fat calories by the number of total calories. For example, if the number of fat grams in a serving is 3, the fat provides 27 (3 x 9) calories. If the total number of calories in the serving is 150, the percentage of fat in the product is 18 (27 ÷ 150 = .18). If you avoid eating any food that

---

A COMPARISON OF SPREADS

Originally margarine was manufactured as a war-time substitute for butter but has now become a product in its own right and spawned many variants that combine butter's taste with margarine's spreadability. The comparison below shows the differences in the nutritional values of four different types of spreads.

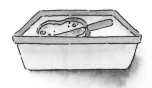

SPREADS THAT ARE VERY LOW IN FAT
Per 100 g: about 273 calories, 25g fat and negligible cholesterol.

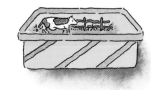

BLENDS OF DAIRY PRODUCTS AND VEGETABLE OILS
Per 100 g: about 739 calories, 81.6 g fat and 225 mg cholesterol.

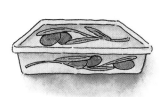

MARGARINES THAT ARE HIGH IN POLYUNSATURATES
Per 100 g: about 739 calories, 81.6g fat and 7 mg cholesterol.

SPREADS WITH AN OLIVE OIL BASE
Per 100 g: about 545 calories, 60 g fat, and negligible cholesterol.

73

WHICH SNACKS ARE HEALTHY?

There are many low-calorie, low-fat snacks that will leave you feeling guilt-free and satisfied. Keep your kitchen stocked with the foods listed below:

▶ *Fruit, fresh or canned with natural juices rather than sugar*

▶ *Rice cakes*

▶ *Fruit, dried, such as raisins, apricots, and figs*

▶ *Breakfast cereals without sugar coatings*

▶ *Low-fat or nonfat yogurt*

▶ *Low-fat or nonfat cheese*

▶ *Raw or blanched vegetables*

▶ *Sorbet*

▶ *Pickles*

▶ *Low-fat crackers*

▶ *Bread sticks*

▶ *Air-popped popcorn*

A HEALTHY TREAT
Raw or lightly blanched vegetables are not only low in fat but also contain filling fiber. To make them even more appealing, serve them with a dip made with low-fat yogurt or cottage cheese mixed with herbs.

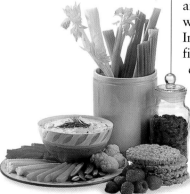

contains more than 30 percent fat per serving, you will remain easily within the limits. However, if you do eat one that is higher, simply balance it with a lower-fat item.

Low-cholesterol foods

Food labels that say "low cholesterol" or "no cholesterol" can be helpful for someone who is watching his cholesterol levels. However, a "low cholesterol" or "no cholesterol" label does not mean that a product will help you lose weight, nor even that it will be better for your health. Of greater value is knowing the amount of saturated fat in a product. If you need to lower your blood cholesterol levels, you should limit foods with a high saturated fat content— whole-milk products, fatty meats, and baked goods made with tropical oils—and increase your intake of cholesterol-lowering foods like oat bran, legumes, and fruits. Olive oil contains monounsaturated fatty acids known to lower cholesterol, but it does have the same number of fat calories as other oils and should be used sparingly.

Sugar and sugar substitutes

Although some types of sugars are regarded by consumers as being healthier than others, all contain the same number of calories per weight and these are empty ones (brown sugar contains insignificant amounts of iron and other minerals). Therefore if you are trying to lose weight or maintain a healthy weight, you should cut down on all sugars, including honey and maple syrup.

The sugar substitutes aspartame and saccharin contain virtually no calories . (Aspartame actually contains the same calories, weight for weight, as sugar, but because it is 60 times sweeter, it can provide a teaspoon's worth of sweetness with one-tenth of a calorie.) As part of a weight-loss program, they are useful for sweetening foods and drinks, but aspartame loses its sweetness when exposed to heat and certain acids. Instead of satisfying a sweet tooth with artificial sweeteners, however, it is more beneficial to change your eating habits to include a variety of healthy, low-sugar foods and naturally sweet foods like fruit. One study on 78,000 women revealed that those who reported using artificial sweeteners gained more weight in a year than nonusers. It's possible that artificial sweeteners actually increase appetite.

Substitutes for forbidden foods

Some health foods are presented as substitutes for so called forbidden foods, giving the impression that eating them will not affect a weight-control program. Frozen yogurt, for example, is no less fattening than ice cream unless it is a low-fat version. It is possible to substitute low-calorie foods for high-calorie versions, however, without compromising on taste. For instance, mayonnaise can be obtained in low-calorie and nonfat types. Sour cream and cream cheese, too, are available in low-fat and nonfat versions that usually stand in nicely for the originals. Heat can affect these last two in unexpected ways, however, so it is better not cook with them .

Check labels and compare brands to make sure you are choosing a product that really makes a difference. Compare total fat content, sugar content, and calories per serving for similar products. If the difference is at least 20 percent, it probably is worth trying.

Try to replace completely those foods that are very high in fat. Yogurt is a useful substitute for almost any form of cream. It can be added to sauces and soups to give a creamy texture (though it should be added at the last minute because it curdles when cooked) and substituted for butter on baked potatoes.

CHAPTER 5

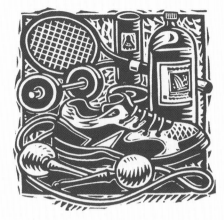

EXERCISE AND YOUR WEIGHT

Exercise, in some form, is a vital part of any weight-control program. Combining careful management of your diet with regular exercise is, without doubt, the most successful way to reach and maintain your ideal weight. Exercise has the added benefit of increasing fitness and general well-being.

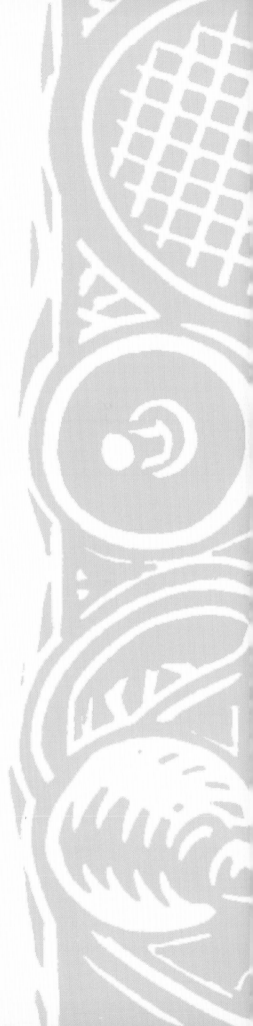

USING EXERCISE TO CONTROL WEIGHT

In the past, the emphasis in weight reduction has been on calorie restriction. Today, however, it is known that weight management is most successful when exercise and diet work hand-in-hand.

If you take in more food energy (calories) than your body requires for general functioning, you will gain weight. The excess energy not used up by your body is converted to fat and stored. If your intake and output of energy are equal, your weight will remain constant. The best long-term solution for weight loss, therefore, is to reduce your energy intake by modifying your diet and simultaneously increase your energy output by doing more exercise.

Dieting alone can be difficult to maintain. You may feel weak and lethargic, if you reduce your food intake too dramatically, and find it difficult to maintain strict control over the food you eat. There is also clinical evidence to support the importance of exercise in weight control: one recent study in the United States, for example, followed the progress of two groups over a period of 12 weeks. One group followed a low calorie diet; the second followed the same diet but carried out an exercise program at the same time. Members of the second group not only were more successful at losing weight in the short term but also did better at maintaining the weight loss. A follow-up after 24 weeks showed that the exercise group had on average regained only 0.4 kg (14 oz) in weight compared with the diet-only group's average weight regain of 1.8 kg (4 lb).

EXERCISE AND WEIGHT LOSS

The body uses energy just to keep itself alive: breathing, making the heart beat, maintaining organ functions, and producing heat all call on energy converted by the body from food. During exercise, additional demands are placed on the body's supply of energy. Different types of physical activity make different energy demands; strenuous exercise like swimming continuously for 20 minutes will burn more energy than walking, for instance. But you can still achieve significant weight loss with only moderate exercise if you do it on a daily basis.

MUSCLE VERSUS FAT

Muscle and fat cells have different cellular structures and functions. Fats, or lipids, are stored as adipose tissue just beneath the skin and around various internal organs and serve as a concentrated source of energy for the body. These cells increase in number and size when a person puts on weight.

THE FAT HIDDEN IN YOUR MUSCLES

Many people do not realize that considerable deposits of fat can be stored around muscle fibers. However, regular aerobic exercise can improve the condition of the muscles, increasing the number of capillaries running through them. This improves the supply of blood carrying oxygen to the muscles. The size and number of mitochondria enzymes (which produce energy) within each individual muscle cell also increase, so that the muscle is able to function much more efficiently.

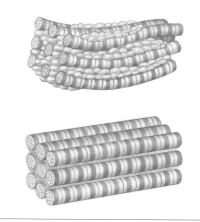

UNEXERCISED MUSCLE
The fibers of unexercised muscle are surrounded by fat deposits and the muscle itself is smaller and less oxygenated than exercised muscle.

EXERCISED MUSCLE
Toned muscle becomes lean and increases in density, with more and larger capillaries and aerobic enzymes, which promote more efficient energy production.

Adipose tissue makes up a larger portion of the total body weight of women than of men (20 to 25 percent of total body weight, compared to 15 to 20 percent for a man). This difference ensures that women have adequate energy stores for reproduction.

Muscle cells are long and slender in structure compared with fat cells, which are round, and are capable of contraction and relaxation to create movement. There are three types of muscles: skeletal, smooth, and cardiac. Skeletal muscles are by far the largest group in the body. Under the body's conscious control, they are activated by the brain to perform various functions like taking a step. Skeletal muscles account for 40 to 45 percent of total body weight. Smooth and cardiac muscles are not under conscious control: they regulate the action of internal organs such as the bowel and heart.

How muscles affect weight

Muscle cells weigh up to three times more than fat cells, which is why a man generally weighs more than a woman of the same height: more of a man's total body weight consists of muscle. Also, it takes more energy (calories) to fuel a muscle cell than a fat cell. Regular exercise will increase the bulkiness of muscles and their demand for fuel. In response, metabolic rate will increase to provide the extra energy needed, by burning more calories, thus helping a person lose weight. A diet-only weight-loss plan can produce unwanted effects on metabolic rate. About 25 percent of the weight lost in a

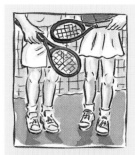

QUICK FITNESS TIP
Avoid planning social occasions around eating out. Instead, invite friends to play a game of tennis or go for a country walk.

COMBINING DIET AND EXERCISE

On a diet-only weight-loss program, you will have to reduce your calorie intake much more significantly in order to lose weight than if you also had an exercise regime. Exercise both burns up calories directly and increases your metabolic rate. Below is a comparison of a day in the life of two different women who both weigh 63.5 kg (140 lb). Justine is moderately active, and so requires about 2,500 calories per day to maintain her weight. In practice, her combination of exercise and careful eating means that her calorie intake is less than this, and she will lose weight. Katie is quite sedentary during the week but more active at weekends; she needs about 2,000 calories per day. As her calorie intake is much higher, she will gain weight unless she makes some lifestyle changes. She also eats far more fat than Justine, and studies show that the amount of fat in the diet is at least as important as the number of calories in determining weight gain and fat deposition.

JUSTINE'S DAY			
FOOD INTAKE	KCAL (FAT)	EXERCISE/ LIFESTYLE	KCALS BURNT
Breakfast – bran flakes, bagel with low-fat spread, coffee with milk and sugar	440 (16 g)	20-min brisk walk to bus	100
2 chocolate chip cookies	97 (5 g)		
Lunch – tuna (in water) salad sandwich, low-fat yogurt, coffee	369 (3.2 g)	30-min brisk walk at lunch	150
Snack – raisins	267 (0.4 g)	20-min brisk walk home	100
Dinner – roast chicken (without skin), baked potato, carrot, broccoli, low-fat ice cream, fruit juice	800 (22 g)		
Snack – banana	95 (0.3 g)		
Bedtime drink – herbal tea	2		
TOTAL	2070 (46.9g)		350

KATIE'S DAY			
FOOD INTAKE	KCAL (FAT)	EXERCISE/ LIFESTYLE	KCALS BURNT
Breakfast – croissant with butter and jam, coffee (milk and sugar)	342 (18 g)	10-min drive to work	16
Doughnut	235 (10 g)		
Lunch – tuna (in oil) salad sandwich, whole-milk yogurt, coffee	497 (13 g)	Lunch at her desk	16
Snack – mixed nuts/raisins	481 (34 g)	10-min drive home	16
Dinner – roast chicken (with skin), baked potato, fried tomato, carrot, broccoli, regular ice cream, 2 glasses of wine	1136 (48 g)		
Snack – chocolate bar	736 (34 g)		
Bedtime drink – cocoa	127 (4.3 g)		
TOTAL	3554 (161.3 g)		48

How to prevent dehydration during exercise

It is vital to keep up your fluid levels during exercise. Becoming dehydrated can affect your ability to use your muscles and even make you physically ill. During an hour's exercise you can lose about a quart of fluid through sweat and in the form of water vapor you breathe out. Be especially careful to keep up your fluid intake when exercising in very hot weather and always take a supply of water with you when doing any exercise at all, even going for a walk. High-energy means high-calorie, so sports drinks are best avoided during a weight-loss plan. Water is the best choice for efficient rehydration without adding calories.

diet-only regime is lean muscle. This means that you will lower your metabolic rate as less and less energy is required and find it harder to lose weight. Because exercise tones your muscles, it can also improve your general appearance, which is ultimately what most dieters are trying to achieve.

Can muscle turn into fat?

Happily, this common fear is a biological impossibility because the cellular composition and functions of muscle and fat are very different (see page 76). If you have been carrying out a regular exercise program for a long time and then stop, your muscles will waste relatively quickly, losing their firmness and tone. They may look like fat (or more precisely, flab), but once you resume exercising your muscles will return to their former tone.

Avoiding overenlarged muscles

Muscles can hypertrophy (enlarge) as a result of excessive and constant demand—for example, from load bearing or resistance exercise like body building and, to a lesser extent, weight lifting. It can also happen in other more general activities such as step aerobics, when they are performed to excess. If muscle size increases but body fat levels have not decreased simultaneously (because you have increased your calorie intake), you might look larger, as layers of fat rest over the muscle, and you would also

ENERGY FOR EXERCISE

To be truly effective, your exercise plan needs to be properly fueled. Not enough fuel or the wrong kind can make you feel prematurely tired. If your diet contains the recommended level of carbohydrates (see page 60) you will be eating enough for most exercise needs. But strenuous or prolonged exercise may require an extra energy boost, such as a banana or other fruit or a baked potato, eaten two hours before. Up to two hours after exercise the body's system of breaking down food into usable energy is at its most efficient, so it is important to refuel with a healthy meal and not high-fat snacks and drinks. The latter cannot be efficiently or completely broken down and will be stored as fat.

weigh more. But remember that it is not so much weight you are trying to control but fat. Weight is easy to measure but it is not always an accurate guide to body fat.

Whatever activity you choose, you can safeguard yourself by introducing a range of exercises that concentrate on different groups of muscles. This is called cross-training and will result in muscle improvement all over. It has the added benefit that variation in activity is less likely to cause injury due to repetitive physical stress, and you are less likely to become bored by always following the same training routine.

THE BEST FUEL FOR EXERCISE

It is widely understood that energy stored in the body is burned off during exercise. The two forms used are carbohydrate (stored as glycogen) and fat. Carbohydrate is the form that the body can use most effectively, especially during sustained, intense periods of activity. Studies have shown that eating more carbohydrates in the days preceding a competition can increase an athlete's ability to perform well. Fat, however, does not improve performance in competition and might even make it worse.

Starting from scratch

There is some evidence that low-intensity exercise (aerobic activity in which breathing is easy, such as walking at a moderate pace)

BURNING OFF CALORIES: *Low-impact Aerobics*

Aerobics is a series of movements and exercises put to music. You can either attend a class or exercise to a home video. It is an ideal way of improving your fitness level with a low risk of injury.

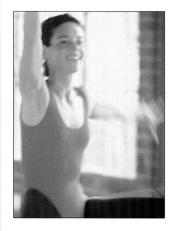

MUSCLE GROUPS BENEFITING
Some classes work all muscle groups while others target specific areas such as legs and the abdomen..

EQUIPMENT
A good pair of training shoes that support your ankles. For women, a sports bra is also recommended.

CALORIES BURNED
8 calories are burned per minute: that's 480 calories in an hour-long session.

performed for long periods can burn up stored fat. Prolonged low-intensity exercise is a sensible way for overweight or very sedentary people to begin exercising. Every activity has a fat burning potential, so if you are trying to lose weight, include more physical effort in your life—for example, walk at least part of the way to work or catch up on some gardening or housework. Choose a form of exercise that can be stepped up gradually to a moderate intensity as you become fitter. Short walks, for instance, can be lengthened, the pace increased, and hills included, as the weeks go by. Visits to your local swimming pool can be treated in the same way.

HOW EXERCISE AFFECTS METABOLISM

The amount of energy that your body uses at rest is determined by your metabolic rate (see page 29). If you can increase the pace of your basic metabolism, you will lose weight more easily, because your body will be calling upon more energy for everything from breathing to running. But it takes a long period of regular exercise to achieve this effect. As discouraging as this may sound, the benefits are still worth the effort. Even light to moderate exercise can prevent the decrease in metabolic rate that would naturally occur if you tried to lose weight by decreasing calories only.

EXERCISING AT THE RIGHT INTENSITY

Once you have achieved a reasonable level of fitness, learning to measure your heart rate will help you assess if your exercise routine is making your body work hard enough.

A target heart rate zone is largely determined by age and fitness levels. To find your maximum heart rate (beats per minute), subtract your age from 220. Multiply this figure by 0.55 and also 0.85 to find a personal range at 55 percent to 85 percent of your maximum. This is the level you should aim for when you train. Your pulse during exercise should at least be up to the lower level but not exceed the higher one, or there may be too much strain on your heart.

Take your pulse (see instructions, right) during and after activity to check that your training is both safe and effective. Working at your maximum is not medically recommended. If the intensity of the activity is low—with a pulse of 55 to 65 percent—the duration should be longer. If the intensity is greater—with a pulse rate between 65 and 85 percent—the duration can be shorter for the same effect. If your Body Mass Index is 30 or over (see page 25), if your resting heart rate is in the poor range (see chart below), or if you have a medical condition, you should consult with a doctor before setting heart rate targets. You may have to start a fitness routine more slowly.

Finding your average pulse rate

Take your pulse (see below) on three separate mornings, immediately after waking, and calculate the average. Resting heart beats per minute are usually between 60 and 80 (lower for men, higher for women). Use the charts on the left to assess your pulse rate.

CHECKING YOUR PULSE RATE

To determine if your exercise routine is efficient, use your pulse rate as a guide. Your resting pulse reflects your true level of fitness. Generally, the lower your pulse rate the fitter you are. Your pulse during exercise tells you how hard your body is working and can be a warning sign if the level is too high to be safe.

RESTING PULSE RATE				
AGE	POOR	FAIR	GOOD	EXCELLENT
MEN				
20–29	86+	70–84	62–68	60 or less
30–39	86+	72–84	64–70	62 or less
40–49	90+	74–88	66–72	64 or less
50+	90+	76–88	68–74	66 or less
WOMEN				
20–29	96+	78–94	72–76	70 or less
30–39	98+	80–96	72–78	70 or less
40–49	100+	80–98	74–78	72 or less
50+	104+	84–102	76–82	74 or less

RECOVERY PULSE RATE AFTER 30 SECONDS				
AGE	POOR	FAIR	GOOD	EXCELLENT
MEN				
20–29	102+	86–100	76–84	74 or less
30–39	102+	88–100	80–86	78 or less
40–49	106+	90–104	82–88	80 or less
50+	106+	92–104	84–90	82 or less
WOMEN				
20–29	112+	94–110	88–92	86 or less
30–39	114+	96–112	88–94	86 or less
40–49	116+	96–114	90–94	88 or less
50+	118+	100–116	92–98	90 or less

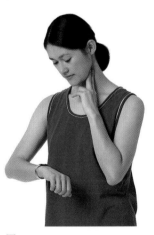

TAKING YOUR PULSE Locate the carotid artery under the jaw using your fingers. Count the beats for 15 seconds and multiply by 4. This is your 1-minute reading.

THE RIGHT EXERCISE

Before introducing more physical activity into your life, give some thought to selecting the right type of exercise and the best routine to suit your age and lifestyle.

Warming-up correctly
A crucial part of every exercise session, warming up prepares your body for exercise by stimulating your cardiovascular system and preparing your muscles.

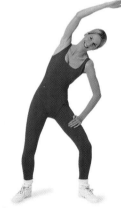

GENTLE STRETCHING
Stretch all the major muscle groups, keeping movements smooth, gentle, and relaxed.

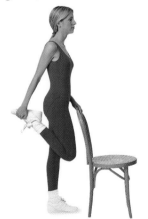

HOLDING THE STRETCH
For maximum benefit hold the stretch for 8 to 10 seconds, always maintaining correct posture.

There are two types of exercise: aerobic and anaerobic. Aerobic exercise is any form of prolonged activity that can be performed continuously for at least 12 minutes and that uses oxygen to provide energy for the muscles. This includes brisk walking, jogging, cycling, swimming, and aerobic dancing (body toning exercises set to music). The latter is either low-impact or high-impact: low-impact exercises tend to be gentler, while high-impact exercises are more jarring to the body, because they involve jumps or running.

Anaerobic exercise consists of short, high-intensity bursts of strenuous activity such as weight lifting or sprinting, in which the heart and lungs cannot meet the oxygen needs of the muscles. Different chemical reactions take place in the body to provide fuel for anaerobic exercise, and exercise cannot be maintained for long periods because the body's refueling system is not as efficient. Aerobic exercise is therefore the best form of activity both for efficient burning of calories and for general health.

STARTING TO EXERCISE

It is important to be realistic when starting an exercise routine. You will do more harm than good if you push yourself too hard at the beginning. Lack of fitness makes your heart less efficient at pumping blood to the muscles during exercise: they won't have enough oxygen to use as fuel and will tire more rapidly, and your reflexes will slow down. This increases the risk of injury.

If you are over 40, have an existing medical condition, have a BMI above 30 (see page 25), or if your resting heart rate is in the poor range (see page 79), it is sensible to have a checkup with your doctor before starting an exercise regimen. Your doctor can check your blood pressure and heart rate, advise you on a suitable level of exer-

cise, and warn against particular forms of exercise that may be inappropriate.

When you first begin to exercise you may experience muscle aches but these will pass as the muscle groups adjust to being used. Warming up the muscles before a workout is important and will help to reduce the likelihood of aches and pains.

There are some warning signs from your body that should not be ignored. Fainting during exercise is a serious danger signal. It suggests a reduced flow of blood to the brain, which could be due to a decrease in blood pressure or a sudden change in the rhythm of your heart. If you experience chest pains or extreme breathlessness, you should see your doctor as soon as possible.

Any increase in your level of activity should be implemented slowly. Adults should build up to 30 minutes or more of low- to moderate-intensity aerobic exercise on at least three days of the week. For example, you could begin with a 10-minute session twice a week, gradually increasing the length of time you perform the exercise and the number of sessions each week.

Low to moderate forms of aerobic exercise include walking, gentle swimming, and gentle cycling. If activities such as

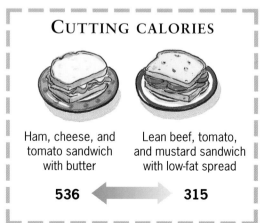

CUTTING CALORIES

Ham, cheese, and tomato sandwich with butter

536

Lean beef, tomato, and mustard sandwich with low-fat spread

315

housework and gardening are sufficiently vigorous and prolonged to raise your heart rate, they would also count as reasonable forms of exercise. Older people may benefit from specially designed low-impact exercise classes held at local community centers and the YMCA. The key to success, however, is that the exercise is performed at least three times a week on a regular basis.

THE BEST TIME TO EXERCISE

Once you begin your new exercise regimen it is important to maintain it, so arrange to exercise at times that fit most readily into your existing lifestyle. For example, if your job is demanding and stressful, consider taking an exercise break in the middle of the day. Not only might this be the most convenient time, but also exercise at this time can help relieve tension, clear your mind, and actually make you more effective in your job for the remainder of the afternoon. If you can find a gym near your workplace, use the exercise bike or the step machine for at least 20 minutes.

With little enough time to fit in both work and social activities, many people cannot even consider exercising in the evening. If your evenings are always busy, consider swimming in the morning before work. It can be a great way to start the day.

If you have a family, look at ways to make the evening a time for family exercise. For instance, could you all go for a bike ride or swim in an indoor pool twice a week? This will not only provide you with useful exercise but also be fun time spent with the family and, in addition, will probably help to give you a good night's sleep. Once you have established the most convenient time to exercise, it is important to do it regularly.

RISKS OF OVER-EXERCISING

Too much exercise is potentially as harmful as too little. Unless the body is given time to recover after each session, the continuous wear can lead to muscle injuries such as strains or tears. Gentle, regular exercise, such as walking, can be performed several times a week but more strenuous exercise, such as a workout at the gym, should be followed by a rest day so that muscles can recover. Erratic bouts of exercise without proper warm-up and cool-down sessions can put unhealthy strain on the heart, particularly in older people.

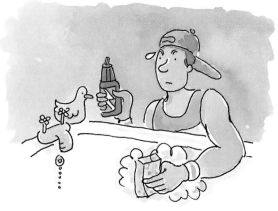

Excessive exercising can also cause more serious health problems. Strenuous workouts in very hot weather may lead to heat exhaustion. Symptoms include dizziness, nausea, and cramps. In serious cases heat stroke can result, and this can be life threatening. To avoid heat exhaustion drink plenty of water before, during, and after exercise. Wear light, comfortable clothing, and in very hot weather, consider exercising early in the morning or later in the evening.

Long-term strenuous exercise for women may also lead to amenorrhea (the cessation of menstruation), by reducing the level of hormones that control the menstrual cycle. If your weight drops substantially below the

continued on page 84

ELBOW GREASE
Housework can burn a surprising number of calories, especially if you put your back into it. Light housework like dusting or vacuuming can burn up to 4 calories per minute. Vigorous activities, like scrubbing the bathtub or moving furniture, can burn between 5 and 7.5 calories per minute.

AEROBIC VERSUS ANAEROBIC EXERCISE

Aerobic exercise needs a steady supply of oxygen to the muscles. It improves cardiovascular fitness and uses up fat stores for energy. Anaerobic exercise is targeted to build muscle rather than improve fitness, and burns only carbohydrate stores, not fat. This type of exercise cannot be sustained for long periods—you can feel exhausted after just a minute or so—and the build-up of lactic acid, a by-product of the anaerobic reaction, can cause muscle pain and fatigue.

AEROBIC EXERCISE
Exercises such as badminton, walking, and swimming are ideal for weight loss.

ANAEROBIC EXERCISE
Anaerobic exercise places more emphasis on building muscle. Activities that fall into this category include weight lifting and ballet lifts.

Skipping

Skipping is one of the best forms of aerobic exercise. It burns off lots of calories, is easy and fun, and can be done at home without expensive equipment. As a low impact exercise, it won't put your knees under stress and will loosen up your shoulders.

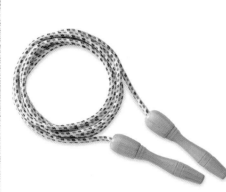

A COMPLETE WORK-OUT
Skipping is a low impact activity because your feet generally stay close to the ground. It is very effective all-around exercise, working especially your back and shoulders and improving the range of movement in your shoulder joints.

Many people don't exercise enough. Some find professionally run classes or gym membership too expensive or it is difficult for them to attend classes regularly. Others may feel embarrassed about exercising in front of other people. But these shouldn't be reasons not to exercise:

the answer is to devise a simple routine that can be practiced at home. Skipping is a useful exercise to increase your total physical fitness. It targets your calves, thighs, and buttocks, and can easily be done at home. All you need is enough room to swing the rope.

WARMING UP AND COOLING DOWN

Begin all forms of exercise with some basic warm-up stretches like the ones shown here. These should last approximately 10 minutes. Use the same stretches to cool down after your exercise session.

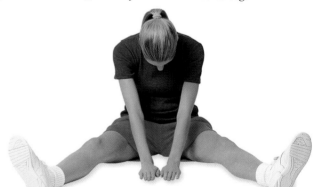

THIGH STRETCH
Lie face down with your stomach in and your hips pressed to the floor. Rest your forehead on your left arm, keeping your head in line with your spine. With knees together, bend your right knee, reaching

back with your right hand to pull your foot toward your buttocks. When you feel tension in the front of your thigh, hold the stretch for 8 to 10 seconds. Repeat with the other leg.

ARM STRETCH
Stand with your back straight, your stomach tucked in, and your hips tilted slightly forward. Your feet should be about hip width apart and your knees slightly bent. Raise your left arm; place your left hand behind your head and between your shoulder blades. Placing your right hand over your left elbow, ease your elbow toward the midline of your body. Keep your head upright and facing forward. Hold the stretch for 8 to 10 seconds. Repeat with the other arm.

GROIN STRETCH
Sit with back straight, legs apart, and stomach pulled in. Start with head up and hands on inner thighs. Bend forward

from the hips and place hands flat on the floor in front of you. Reach forward until you feel tension in the groin. Keep your toes pointing up.

BUYING THE RIGHT ROPE

The most important thing when buying a skipping rope is to make sure that it is the right length. Also, select a hard-wearing, heavy rope.

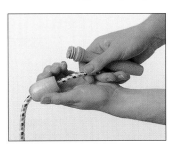

SHORTENING THE ROPE
It is usually possible to adjust the length if the rope is too long. Check before you buy.

MEASURING UP
Stand with both feet on the center of the rope and pull up the ends. The handles should reach to your armpits. It is advisable to measure this with string first so that you purchase a long enough rope.

BUILDING UP A REGIME

Many people assume that because skipping is a popular game for children, it cannot be a strenuous enough exercise for adults. But in practice, skipping is a lot harder than it looks.

A regular skipping routine will help you develop your fitness coordination and agility. Skipping also makes an excellent addition to a cross-training program, in which a variety of aerobic and resistance activities—such as skipping and weight lifting—are combined to create a complete cardiovascular workout to achieve all-round fitness.

INTRODUCING A ROUTINE
If you have not skipped for some time, you may find a normal training level too hard. To build up stamina, skip initially for 2 minutes, or if this is too much, for 30 to 40 skips, and then rest for 30 seconds. Repeat twice. At each subsequent session reduce every rest interval by 5 seconds, until you have eliminated all of them.

STARTING A REGIME
You should now be ready to begin a formal training regimen, but this, too, should be introduced gradually. Start with a 3-minute skipping session once a week; then graduate to a 4-minute session twice a week; then a 5-minute session twice a week, building up over 10 sessions to three 20-minute sessions a week.

SKIPPING FOR BEGINNERS

Wearing loose, comfortable clothing and training shoes, begin to skip. Try to keep your shoulders relaxed and your upper arms close to your body. Use your wrists, not your whole arms, to turn the rope and try to keep them as low as possible. Keep your back straight and your stomach pulled in.

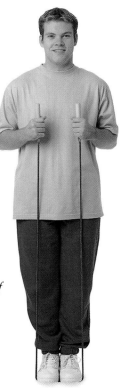

ROCKING SKIP
This is the easiest type of skipping, and because you are half running rather than jumping, it does not require as much energy. At first, step each time with the same foot leading, then try alternating the leading foot. To avoid strain, keep your feet within 2.5 cm (1 in) of the ground and your knees slightly bent to absorb the impact. Keep your head upright, in line with your spine.

JUMPS
As your fitness level increases, begin adding jumps with both feet together. To avoid boredom, you could try some variations such as hopping on one foot, then the other. Again, make sure you do not jump too high. If you keep your feet in fairly close contact with the ground, you will minimize the chance of strain and will more likely keep jumping for a longer time.

THE STEP TEST

This simple test enables you to assess your aerobic endurance and gives you an idea of how fit you really are and what level of intensity your exercise program should be. It is also a useful guide to how your fitness is progressing, once your exercise routine has been established.

If your resting heart rate is in the poor range (see page 79) do not attempt the test and seek advice from your doctor. Before you start the test, carry out a 10-minute stretching session to avoid straining yourself. Find a secure step not more than 20 to 25 cm (8 to 10 inches) high, stand approximately 30 cm (12 inches) away from it, and do the test (see right). Check your results against the recovery rate chart on page 79. If you fall in the poor to fair range, you should start an exercise program very gently.

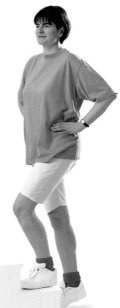

1 *Keep your back straight and stomach in. Step up and down—leading first with the right foot up, then the left up, then right down and so on—as fast as is comfortable for three minutes.*

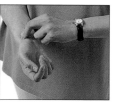

2 *Rest for 30 seconds, and then take your pulse.*

CHARTING PROGRESS
Keeping a record of your exercise regimen will help you measure your progress. Include details of when you exercised, what kind of exercise you performed and for how long, your pulse before and after, and your weight. Over a period of a few months of regular exercise you will see an improvement in your resting and recovery heart rates. Avoid weighing yourself too often, as daily fluctuations can be misleading.

normal body weight for your height this may also lead to amenorrhea. Consult your doctor if you miss three or more periods.

SETTING UP YOUR OWN EXERCISE PROGRAM

The first step in setting up your own exercise program is to find out how fit you are now. Your resting pulse rate already provides some indication of this, but you can also test your endurance by performing the step test (see above). Once your general fitness level is established, you can begin introducing regular exercise at the correct level. If you are not very fit, it is important to begin slowly, gradually building up the intensity of the exercise.

While general aerobic exercise will burn calories, you should also consider additional exercises to improve the muscle tone of specific areas of the body. For example, if you feel that your stomach is too flabby, consider doing abdominal exercises such as sit-ups to strengthen and flatten the stomach and abdominal muscles.

Remember that in order to lose weight, you should consume the right number of calories for your levels of activity (see charts, page 49), which are delivered in a well balanced diet (see page 51).

Exercising for body shape

People who usually follow diet-only weight loss programs will notice that when they add an exercise routine, their muscles strengthen and tone at the same time as their bodies are shedding fat. This produces a much healthier-looking end result, particularly for older women who can sometimes look gaunt and unwell after losing a lot of weight on a diet-only regime.

Because exercise strengthens and tones muscles, it can also be used successfully as a way to give a more defined body shape to people who want to actually gain weight. Concentrating on strength exercises such as lifting weights, is probably the best form of exercise for toning and adding bulk to all the major muscle groups.

DATE	TYPE OF EXERCISE	SESSION DETAILS	RESTING HEART RATE	RECOVERY HEART RATE	STEP TEST RESULTS	WEIGHT (kg)
2 Feb	Skipping	10 mins	84	106	100	63.5
2 Feb	Brisk walk	30 mins	–	–	–	–
3 Feb	Swimming	40 mins	84	104	–	–
3 Feb	Exercises	10 mins	–	–	–	–
5 Feb	Bicycle ride	40 mins	83	108	–	–
5 Feb	Exercises	10 mins	–	–	–	–
2 Mar	Jogging	25 mins	79	100	96	61.5

MAKING EXERCISE A HABIT FOR ALL AGES

Once you have reached your target weight, exercise should remain an important part of your daily life. If your lifestyle changes, you can adapt your exercise plan accordingly.

Getting and keeping fit is essential at any age, but staying with an exercise program for an extended period can be difficult. It can help to get friends and family interested in sharing your goals.

MOTIVATING AND ENCOURAGING CHILDREN TO EXERCISE

Studies have shown an alarming increase in obesity in children. Encouraging children to exercise is the best way to prevent excessive weight gain and to keep them healthy.

You can begin by setting a good example yourself. It is hard to persuade your child to play outside instead of watching television, if you spend most of your own leisure time in front of the set. Investing in bikes and going on regular family bicycle rides can be a great exercise plan. Taking your children on walks to the stores and walking with them to school rather than using the car are also good ways to establish positive habits.

Encourage children in any aptitude they may show for a particular sport and work around problems that may prevent them from taking part. For example, an asthmatic child may have difficulty breathing while exercising, but increased fitness can actually improve asthma. In consultation with your doctor, a suitable routine can be developed. Swimming has been shown to cause exercise-induced asthma less often than other sports, and because most children love playing in water, it's a great way to introduce them to exercise. Increasing your child's fitness outside of school may also help him feel more confident about joining in school sports and other activities.

Making exercise fun is the best way to encourage it. If your children feel intimidated by the pressure of team sports, explore other exercise options with them. For example, orienteering, in which children learn map-reading skills while hiking, may suit a

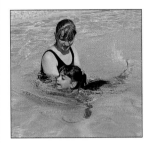

A CONFIDENCE BOOST
Swimming is excellent exercise for people of all ages. By introducing your children to the sport at an early age, you can prevent them from developing a fear of water. Once they become competent swimmers, they can amuse themselves in a pool while you swim some laps.

EXERCISE AND ASTHMA

In some people exercise can bring on the wheezing and breathlessness of an asthma attack. This is because exercise increases the flow of air through small airways in the lungs (called bronchioles), causing irritation and narrowing of the airway lining and restricting the flow of oxygen. Exercising in a warm, humid environment reduces the chance of irritation, therefore, swimming is a good form of exercise for asthmatics. Using a bronchodilator just before exercising also helps lower the risk of an asthma attack. Exercise should be avoided in cold or dry conditions.

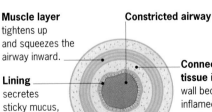

Open airway

Muscle layer tightens up and squeezes the airway inward.

Lining secretes sticky mucus, which blocks the already narrow airway.

Constricted airway

Connective tissue in the wall becomes inflamed and swells, which narrows the airway further.

HEALTHY BRONCHIOLE
This cross-section of a normal bronchiole shows the rings of muscle and connective tissue in a relaxed, unconstricted state.

ASTHMATIC BRONCHIOLE
During an asthma attack, a bronchodilator is used to relax and open the airway. Seek medical attention if it fails to have this effect.

more introverted youngster. Or if your child loves music, sign her up for ballet, jazz dance, or aerobics classes, or let her wear a personal stereo while joining in the family walk, if this increases motivation.

Encourage young people to participate in exercises that are appropriate for their ages. During early childhood the focus should be on fun games and activities that develop the basic movement skills of running, balancing, jumping, kicking, and throwing. Between the ages of 6 and 12 more emphasis can be given to areas where a child shows a particular talent.

Most experts agree that the same level of exercise intensity and frequency advised for average adults should be applied to children—that is, low- to moderate-intensity exercise undertaken for 30 minutes three to four times a week. The responses of children to exercise are similar to those of adults, but children generally recover more quickly. However, since they cannot hold as much oxygen in their lungs as grown-ups can, they are unable to match an adult's ability to endure a prolonged workout. Exercising during very hot weather can also be a problem. Because they have lower sweat rates, their bodies are less able to cool quickly through evaporation. It is therefore important that children avoid exercise in the middle of the day during hot weather and that they drink plenty of fluids.

EXERCISING AS YOU GET OLDER

Maintaining an exercise plan as you age has important benefits. Exercising can prevent middle-age spread, slow down the stiffening of joints, and relieve other age-related illnesses such as osteoporosis.

There is no age limit on exercise, and clinical evidence suggests that there need not be a severe decline in fitness with age. In an experiment conducted in a nursing home in 1995 by a specialist in Massachusetts, 10 men aged 86 to 96, all of whom had ortho-

DID YOU KNOW?

In 1987, at the age of 67 years and 241 days, Australian swimmer Bertram Clifford Batt became the oldest person ever to swim the English Channel: a distance of some 21 miles (34 km). The swim was completed in a time of 18 hours, 37 minutes.

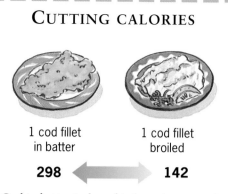

CUTTING CALORIES

1 cod fillet in batter	1 cod fillet broiled
298	**142**

Cod in batter is deep-fried, so that extra fat comes from both the batter and the oil.

pedic difficulties, volunteered to take up weight training. They showed significant gains in leg muscle strength and size. In 1988, Dr. William Evans in the United States, discovered that men ranging in age from 60 yo 72 years were able to increase their muscular strength by 200 percent with regular exercise and weight training.

It is wise to consult your doctor before beginning an exercise program. In the beginning, avoid very strenuous activities and concentrate on relaxing, gentle forms of movement. Low-impact exercises such as swimming and walking are the most suitable, as these place the least stress on joints. Also, low intensity exercise, which has a lower risk of injury and cardiorespiratory stress, is generally more appropriate.

Exercises should be tailored to any medical conditions. For example, people who suffer degenerative joint disease will do best with non-weight-bearing activities such as stationary cycling or water exercises. On the other hand, women who are susceptible to or show signs of osteoporosis should be doing weight-bearing exercises to increase their bone density. Suitable ones include low-impact aerobics, walking, stair climbing, and weight lifting. Anyone who has high blood pressure, heart disease, or arthritis should avoid weight-lifting, as these exercises can place excessive strain on the body.

Because the body's thermal control system becomes less efficient in old age, exerting the body during extreme weather conditions should be avoided. It's best to exercise in winter during the warmest part of the day and vice versa in summer. For the same reason dehydration can also be a problem, and drinking plenty of fluids is essential.

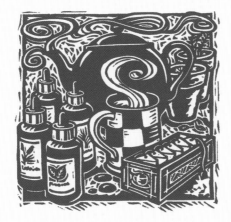

CHAPTER 6

NATURAL THERAPIES AND YOUR WEIGHT

The self-regulating processes of a healthy body will usually keep your weight in the right range, but these can sometimes get out of kilter. Natural therapies work gently on body chemistry, physiology, and emotional harmony, and, when combined with an improved diet and an increase in physical activity, can be used to help restore and maintain a healthy weight.

MIND AND BODY

Natural therapies can help you achieve the goal of successful weight control by working with your physical and mental resources to stimulate the body's built-in self-regulating abilities.

Natural therapies are those that use the resources of nature to promote normal healthy bodily functions. There are many different approaches, but all are aimed primarily at encouraging the body's inherent mechanisms of self-repair.

Some, such as acupuncture and acupressure, have their origins in antiquity but are applied today with more precision in the light of modern knowledge. Others, such as homeopathy and psychotherapy, were developed in recent times by pioneering physicians. Which ones are most appropriate for you will depend on the underlying cause of your body's imbalance.

USING NATURAL THERAPIES

Techniques like meditation focus on mental and emotional well-being, while others such as naturopathy are aimed more at physiological functions, for instance, modulating body chemistry by correcting nutritional imbalances or stimulating certain responses by physical means. For example, a naturopath might recommend changes to your diet and suggest supplements or herbs to assist the metabolism.

Herbal medicine might be helpful when a specific organ, such as the liver, is malfunctioning and interfering with the efficient working of the digestive system. Homeopathy, on the other hand, works on both physical and mental levels, with remedies chosen according to the individual's particular temperament as well as symptoms.

Therapies such as acupuncture and reflexology make use of the network of nerve and energy pathways within the body to regulate mental and physical imbalances.

No shortcuts

Many natural therapies can make a positive contribution to weight control but no single system can do everything. Some are more effective in combination; for example, when herbal medicines are used to reinforce dietary measures. By incorporating the positive suggestions of hypnotherapy or the insights of counseling into your program, you can adopt a much broader approach. These therapies help you deal with problems such as food cravings, depression, and anxiety, any of which may be preventing you from reaching your weight goals.

Natural therapies can help you get the most from your weight-control regimen, because they are tailored to your individual needs. Whatever approach you choose, it is essential to combine it with a well-planned diet and a suitable exercise program.

ENERGY CENTERS

Developed in ancient India, ayurvedic medicine focuses on seven energy centers (chakras) between the crown of the head and the base of the spine, which are believed essential to health. Each chakra is linked to one or more body parts:

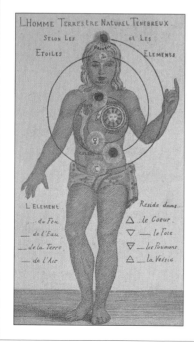

▶ *Sahasrara (crown): whole being.*

▶ *Ajna (brow): brain.*

▶ *Vishuddi (throat): lungs, throat.*

▶ *Anahata (heart): arms, heart.*

▶ *Manipura (solar plexus): small intestine, liver, stomach, spleen.*

▶ *Svadisthana (sacral): reproductive organs, kidneys, bladder.*

▶ *Muladhara (base): large intestine.*

EAST MEETS WEST
This illustration showing the seven chakras comes from the Theosophica Practica. *It was published by the Theosophical Society, formed in France in 1875 by Helena Blavatsky to introduce Eastern philosophy to the West.*

Reflexology

Reflexology is an ancient healing art that therapists believe can restore health to organs of the body. It can play an important part in a weight-control program by improving body functions such as digestion and metabolism.

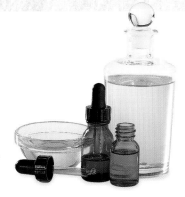

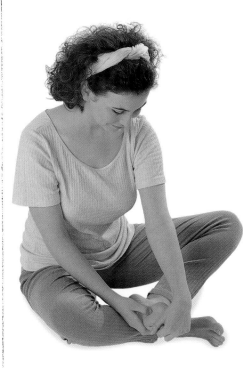

Reflexology is based on the belief that every organ in the body corresponds to zones on the sides and soles of the feet, and that massaging the zones will promote health.

To use the technique on yourself, sit comfortably on a chair or bed with your feet bare; bend one knee and grasp one foot with both hands.

Using the index or middle fingers, knead the zones shown below; spend up to one minute on each area. If a spot is tender, work gently until the discomfort eases. Work on all the relevant zones for a few minutes every day or, if you prefer, select two or three of the zones you feel are the most important for daily attention, treating others once or twice a week as added tonics.

ADDED BENEFIT
Using essential oils as you massage will increase the benefits to the organs.

USING ESSENTIAL OILS

Aromatherapy uses essential oils extracted from flowers, plants, trees, and spices for their antiseptic and anti-bacterial properties and the therapeutic effects of their scents. As feet are sensitive, the oils should never be used straight from the bottle. They should be diluted —about one drop of aromatherapy oil to every 10 ml (2 tsp) of base oil such as jojoba, sweet almond, or wheat germ.

THUMB WALKING

The most fundamental technique in reflexology, thumb walking, takes practice to perfect. Your thumb may be sore at first until it has gained strength.

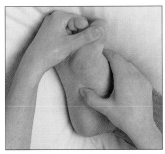

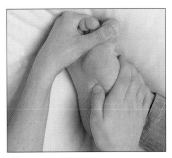

1 *Press the ball of your thumb into the instep of your foot, then walk the thumb up toward the toes by slightly bending and unbending it at its joint.*

2 *As you walk your thumb forward, keep it in gentle contact with the skin. Don't straighten the thumb completely or you will cover areas too quickly.*

ZONES TO TREAT

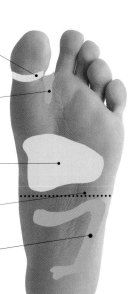

Thyroid – on the soles in a narrow band around the "neck" of the big toes. Use essential oil of sage here, as it is a good general metabolism stimulant.

Lymphatic system – between the first and second toes on the tops and soles of the feet. Rub in juniper or lemon oil—both of which are known for their detoxifying properties.

Stomach – the inner square inch on the sole of the left foot between the ball and "waistline." Use fennel, cardamom, or peppermint oil to ease indigestion and upset stomach.

Waistline

Large intestine – A line of 2.5 to 5 cm (1 to 2 in) up the outer side of each sole and across the center just below the "waistline." Rose, rosemary, and marjoram are good essential oils for this area; they help ease bowel movements.

THERAPIES FOR YOUR BODY

Natural therapies, which make use of herbs, flowers, foods, and water, can play a part in helping you reach your weight goals, especially when used in conjunction with a diet and exercise plan.

Herbal drinks
Health food stores sell dried herbs for use in infusions. These are usually made by pouring hot water over 1 or 2 heaping teaspoons in a cup and leaving it to steep for 10 to 15 minutes. Such teas can be drunk up to 3 or 4 times a day.

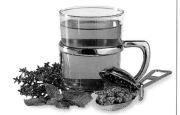

PREPARING AN INFUSION
You can prepare your own herbal drinks at home using fresh herbs— a handful of mint, thyme, or parsley leaves, for example.

Although they are diverse in their approaches, natural therapists are united in their belief that health is dependent on the interaction of body and mind and that it is important to treat a person as a whole, searching out the underlying causes of an illness or condition, rather than just treating symptoms.

HERBALISM

One of the oldest and most universal forms of medical care is the use of plant preparations—roots, stems, leaves, flowers, and seeds—internally or on the skin. Modern phytotherapy (medical herbalism) uses plants to treat various illnesses and diseases as well as to promote general health and well-being. Herbalists use a whole plant or specific parts, rather than a drug derived from it, because they believe as yet unidentified compounds in the plant may play an important role in the therapeutic effect.

As part of a weight-control program, herbal medicines can have positive influences on the body's effective functioning. Some herbal treatments assist removal of toxins by promoting sweating (a cleansing function of the skin) or urination (a cleansing of internal waste fluids). Other herbs have properties that stimulate bodily functions that are not working effectively.

Psyllium, the seeds of the plantain species, *Plantago psyllium*, and an ingredient in many over-the-counter laxatives, has been found to assist in weight loss if taken before meals. In an Italian study, dieters who were given 3 grams in water 30 minutes before each meal lost more weight than a control group that did not receive the preparation.

If you choose to use herbal remedies, you should seek the advice of a medical herbalist, who can tailor combinations of herbs to your particular needs. For example, the thyroid gland—which regulates the body's metabolism—is dependent on iodine salts for its effectiveness, and kelp (see box below) can supply these.

As with any medication, it is important not to exceed the recommended dosage of herbal medicines and to stop the treatment if there is any sign of an allergic reaction.

THE PROPERTIES OF KELP

Kelp, another name for many species of seaweed, has been used for over 200 years as a tonic for hypothyroidism (see page 34). Its high iodine content stimulates thyroid production, stabilizing metabolism. Kelp may also help people who have hypothyroidism lose weight by promoting the faster burning of calories. (Anyone with an overactive thyroid or allergy to iodine should avoid taking kelp.)

A USEFUL SUPPLEMENT
Kelp is available in powder and tablet form from most health food stores. If your thyroid function is normal, kelp will not aid weight loss but will still provide useful amounts of iodine, vitamins, and minerals.

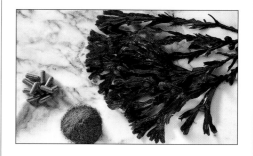

CUTTING CALORIES

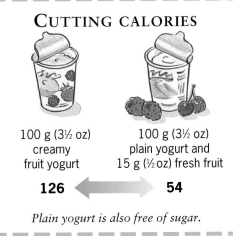

100 g (3½ oz)
creamy
fruit yogurt

126

100 g (3½ oz)
plain yogurt and
15 g (½ oz) fresh fruit

54

Plain yogurt is also free of sugar.

HOMEOPATHY

Homeopathy was founded by the German physician and chemist Samuel Hahnemann in the early 19th century. Today, more than 2,000 homeopathic remedies are in use, derived from a range of plant, animal, and mineral sources. While herbal medicines work directly on the physiology of digestion and other bodily functions, homeopathic remedies influence health more subtly by stimulating the body's powers of self-healing.

The theory behind homeopathy is that "like cures like." According to this idea, a substance that produces certain symptoms in a healthy person can cure a sick person who shows the same symptoms. Because large amounts of a substance can cause many side effects, each medicinal substance is repeatedly diluted by a special process called potentization, until there is no trace of the active ingredient remaining that can be detected by normal chemical analysis.

Homeopaths maintain that the greater the dilution of a remedy the more powerful it becomes and the more carefully it must be matched to the symptoms and characteristics of the patient. These high potency remedies are, therefore, best prescribed by a qualified practitioner. Homeopathic medicines in low potencies are quite safe, and many of them are widely available in both pharmacies and health food stores, either as single remedies or in combinations for particular health needs.

Selecting the right remedy

At a consultation with a homeopath you will be asked a variety of questions ranging well beyond those that seem relevant to your weight problem. Your response to environmental changes and foods, your sleeping habits, temperament, and many other factors can all help the practitioner select the most appropriate treatment. Having chosen one or more remedies, he will prescribe these in a suitable potency (dilution), usually made up in tablet form to be dissolved in water or under the tongue.

Because the active ingredient in a homeopathic medicine has been greatly diluted, it is

FLOWER REMEDIES FOR MIND AND MOOD

Bach flower remedies combine theories of homeopathy and herbal medicine. They are named after their originator, Dr Edward Bach (1886–1936), who believed that certain flowers found in the European countryside can help lessen such negative emotional states as fear, impatience, timidity, grief, or lack of motivation. As research has shown a link between emotional states and food cravings, Bach flower remedies may assist in tackling the emotional issues that are often the root cause of overeating.

The remedies are prepared by distilling freshly picked flowers and other plant parts in bowls of spring water that are left in direct sunlight. They are sold in many pharmacies and health food stores.

Some of the following remedies may be of benefit to people with weight problems:

▶ *Hornbeam – relieves weariness/mental fatigue.*

▶ *Centaury – increases willpower.*

▶ *Chestnut bud – helps to avoid repetition of mistakes, such as impulsive eating.*

▶ *Wild oat – can be a catalyst for change, helping you to make clear decisions.*

▶ *Pine – may help people who tend to reproach themselves.*

HOW MUCH TO TAKE
To make the standard dosage add 2 drops of the remedy to 30 ml (1 fl oz) of water; take 4 drops of this mixture orally four times a day.

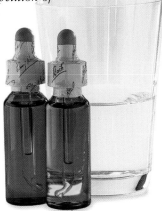

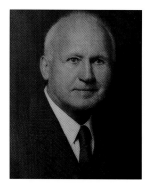

NATURAL PIONEER
German-born Benedict Lust began using the term "naturopathy" in the U.S. in 1902. The term described his vision for the future of natural medicine: a fusing of a diverse range of therapies that include herbal medicine, homeopathy, and nutritional therapy.

easily neutralized by strong tasting or strongly aromatic substances such as spicy foods, alcohol, tobacco, tea, coffee, and toothpaste. For this reason you will be instructed to take medicines well apart from mealtimes, drinks, and brushing your teeth.

Homeopathic remedies that may be beneficial as part of a weight-control program include calcium carbonate, which can reduce water retention, and *Thyroidinum,* which can help combat cravings for sweet foods.

NATUROPATHY

Naturopathy is a system of medicine that encourages people to take considerable responsibility for their own health. It is based on the principle that diseases are the result of incorrect living habits, particularly poor diet. These bad habits result in the accumulation of toxic waste materials that interfere with the body's normal processes.

A naturopath offers advice about various aspects of health care, based on a thorough discussion and medical examination. The treatment will revolve around nutritional changes, supported by physical measures to stimulate metabolism by encouraging the proper functioning of the skin, lungs, bowels, and kidneys, which are responsible for removing waste from the body.

There are many types of diet regimens a naturopath might recommend, depending on your constitution, age, and health history. These may include fasting and cleansing diets, which, along with most other strategies that are advised, can be carried out at home as long as you carefully follow the guidelines provided by the practitioner. Some diets may be combined with hydrotherapy techniques. A naturopath might also prescribe enzyme preparations, herbs, or supplements to assist the digestion and improve the metabolism.

The use of hydrotherapy

Many naturopaths employ hydrotherapy, the healing techniques using water, as part of their treatment. Some methods, such as hot and cold compresses, friction rubs, and seaweed baths can be done at home (see right).

Various forms of hydrotherapy may be recommended to promote more efficient functioning of the skin. The skin is an important organ that has the ability to absorb certain substances—for instance the oils of aromatherapy—in addition to its vital function of eliminating toxic waste products through perspiration. It is also connected by nerve pathways to internal organs such as the liver and kidneys. Therefore stimulation of the skin can have many positive benefits on overall health. A body that is functioning more efficiently will also enhance your weight-control plan.

Residential care

There are a number of centers in North America where residential treatment based on naturopathic principles is given under medical supervision. These clinics provide meals prepared with healthful, low-fat ingredients, plus massage, reflex therapies, exercise regimens, and hydrotherapy, in which more sophisticated equipment for baths, sprays, and steam rooms are used than are normally available in the home. These centers are often in pleasant surroundings, and patients can stay for a week or more to detoxify and shed surplus weight, while learning how to continue a healthier life-style once they have returned home.

Pathway to health

Hydrotherapy techniques that can be of help to people with weight problems include hot and cold compresses, friction rubs, and seaweed baths.

Hot and cold compresses help stimulate blood flow to internal organs such as the stomach and liver. Soak a towel in hot water, wring it out, and apply it to the upper abdominal area for about 3 minutes; then apply one soaked in cold water for 1 minute.

A friction rub stimulates blood circulation, boosts the immune system, and helps the skin shed dead cells. After a hot bath or shower, soak a loofah in cold water and give the body a firm rub down.

A seaweed bath—soaking for 20 to 30 minutes in a hot bath to which seaweed extract has been added—induces perspiration and the uptake of natural iodine and other mineral compounds. Iodine helps stimulate the thyroid gland. Avoid this procedure if you have hyperthyroidism.

The Overeater

The urge to overeat may arise for a number of reasons, both physical and emotional. Metabolic imbalances can create cravings for inappropriate foods or periods of abnormal hunger that may, in turn, affect physical and mental energy. An approach that includes improvements in diet and addresses the underlying psychological factors is essential.

Walter, a 43-year-old marketing manager, was recently warned about his weight during a routine check-up for an insurance policy. His weight and blood pressure have been steadily creeping up and he now realizes that as he ages, he can no longer indulge in high-fat business meals and between-meal snacks as he has in the past. Previously, whenever he tried any form of slimming diet, he became tired and irritable, his hunger increased, and inevitably he reverted to eating unsuitable foods and regained any weight he had lost. Walter is concerned that his rising weight is beginning to affect his health. His primary care physician has suggested that a naturopath might be able to help.

WHAT SHOULD WALTER DO?

After a thorough examination and blood and sweat tests, which revealed shortages of minerals and trace elements that help control levels of fat and cholesterol, the naturopath gave Walter specific advice about his diet.

Walter needs to eat well-balanced meals that sustain his metabolism for longer periods, and remove the need for unhealthy snacks, while also reducing his calorie intake. Low-fat munchies, raw vegetables, and fresh fruit should replace fatty and sugary snacks.

The naturopath explained to Walter how he might benefit his body with his mind (see page 96) and suggested the use of simple hydrotherapy at home (see page 92).

Action Plan

DIET
Eat more fruits and vegetables and include more low-fat protein and complex carbohydrates in meals for sustained energy.

EMOTIONAL HEALTH
Use visualization and meditation to focus on weight-loss goals and improve motivation.

HEALTH
After a morning shower or bath, use a loofah loaded with cold water to rub the skin briskly. This stimulates blood circulation and improves the effectiveness of the kidneys, liver, and lungs.

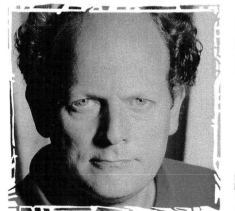

DIET
Insufficient energy from the right kind of food can lead to frequent snacking and overeating.

EMOTIONAL HEALTH
A negative attitude to dieting can lead to failure in weight-control plans. Walter has to believe that his weight goals are achievable to succeed.

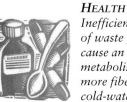

HEALTH
Inefficient elimination of waste products can cause an imbalance in metabolism. Eating more fiber and using cold-water hydrotherapy may help overcome this.

HOW THINGS TURNED OUT FOR WALTER

By eating regular meals based on healthy eating principles, Walter began to feel more energetic and lost his tendency to snack during the day. The naturopath prescribed chromium supplements to aid in glucose metabolism. His cold friction rub in the morning braced him for the day ahead. He started an exercize routine and used visualization to picture himself getting slimmer. As he lost weight and felt better, his ability to concentrate improved.

THERAPIES FOR ENERGY BALANCING

Eastern therapies like acupuncture are based on the belief that any health problem can be improved by balancing the flow of energy through the body's network of energy pathways.

Many therapies aim to restore good health by treating imbalances in the nerve and energy pathways within the body. Reflexology, for example, can be used to aid relaxation and help you prepare your state of mind before beginning a weight-control program.

ACUPUNCTURE

Acupuncture is a form of therapy in which fine needles are applied to acupoints on the body. This network of points lies along a series of channels, or meridians, situated just beneath the skin, and these channels are connected by internal pathways to the major organs. The whole network, which is distinct from the nerves, blood vessels, and lymph channels, makes up an energy system that is believed to regulate all bodily functions. Acupoints are identified by their meridian names—usually that of an associated organ—and a number.

There is some scientific evidence to support acupuncture. It is known that applying needles to acupoints on the skin causes the body to release endorphins, the "feel-good" hormones. While this might account for some of the benefits achieved by acupuncture, it cannot explain other metabolic changes that a qualified practitioner is often able to initiate.

Acupuncture may help to tackle weight problems by improving general well-being, overcoming fatigue, harmonizing digestive functions, reducing tension and anxiety, regulating fluid balance, and controlling the tendency for food cravings.

ACUPRESSURE

It is probable that acupuncture developed out of an older system known as acupressure, or shiatsu. Acupressure also involves acupoints but, as the name suggests, uses pressure rather than needles. It is believed that regular massage of acupoints may act as a tonic to the organs or functions with which they are connected.

Acupressure is best carried out with the tip of the thumb or middle finger or with a rounded device such as a pen top. To stimulate a particular organ or part of the body, apply slow steady pressure and gentle circular kneading movements to the relevant acupoint for one to two minutes at a time. A calming and sedating effect is achieved by sustaining firm, deep, pressure for a longer period—at least two or three minutes.

TREATING CRAVINGS WITH EAR THERAPY

Auricular, or ear, acupuncture is a specialized therapy based on the principle that points on the outer ear relate to each of the major organs. The pattern formed by these points is believed to mirror the position of a fetus in the womb.

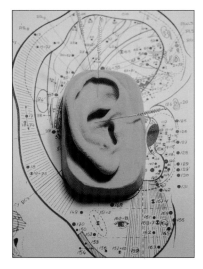

EAR ACUPUNCTURE
Auricular acupuncture uses 120 points on the ear to regulate all other parts of the body. Tiny press needles are inserted by the practitioner and left there under a waterproof plaster for up to two weeks. The patient is instructed to press on the needles several times a day; pressure is barely felt. Practitioners believe that stimulation of the points connected with the digestive organs can help to control addictive tendencies such as food cravings.

ACUPRESSURE FOR WEIGHT CONTROL

Acupressure may help control weight by freeing blocked energy channels and so restoring the healthy functioning of the digestive organs. To stimulate one of the pressure points below, simply apply slow, steady pressure with the thumb or middle finger. Maintain pressure for 20 seconds and release for 10. Repeat this process up to a maximum time of 3 minutes on each point and practice daily.

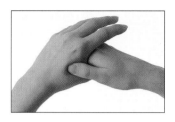

PRESSURE POINT LI 4
To improve bowel function, apply pressure to the back of the hand in the soft flesh between the thumb and index finger.

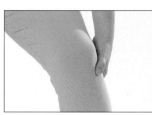

PRESSURE POINT ST 36
To stimulate digestion and metabolism, apply pressure four finger widths below the knee, toward the outside of the shin bone.

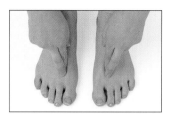

PRESSURE POINT LIV 3
To stimulate the function of the liver, apply pressure to the foot in the angle between the first and second metatarsal bones.

Before selecting the appropriate points, a practitioner of acupuncture or acupressure will make a careful assessment of a patient's needs, using the principles of traditional Chinese medicine, or TCM. This determines the balance of energy flow or evidence of sluggishness in particular parts of the body.

A blockage in the abdominal area, for example, can prevent proper digestive function, causing excess energy to flow upward and leading to heat or flushing in the head or face. In this case, the practitioner will select acupoints principally on the arms, legs, and abdomen.

At the other extreme, energy depletion can lead to fluid retention. In this situation, the practitioner may apply heat to the acupoints by burning an herb called moxa. This technique, called moxibustion, is an invaluable part of TCM that may assist the overweight individual. The treatment increases the general energy and efficiency of the digestive organs and improves metabolism, thereby benefiting any patient who is undergoing a diet and exercise program.

REFLEXOLOGY

There are many areas on the surface of the body that have special points, called reflex points, or zones, that correspond to internal organs. One of the most accessible areas with reflex zones is on the soles of the feet. In the 1930s Eunice Ingham, a New York therapist, rediscovered a system of connecting reflex foot zones to the rest of the body, which she called reflexology. This system had also been known to the ancient Chinese and Egyptians. Ingham found that by massaging tender areas of the feet she could influence the organs connected with them.

The foot zones occupy large areas of the soles, particularly where larger organs like the liver are concerned, so they are relatively easy to locate and manipulate (see page 89).

BURNING OFF CALORIES: *Squash*

A very intense game, squash sharpens the reflexes and demands high energy expenditure and concentration. A good cardiovascular exercise, it will improve endurance, agility, and strength.

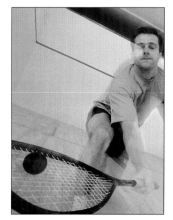

MUSCLE GROUPS BENEFITING
Legs, lower torso, and arm muscles are all utilized during a game.

EQUIPMENT
A court, partner, and racquets and squash balls are required. Light, comfortable clothing is most suitable.

CALORIES BURNED
Playing squash burns about 10 calories a minute (600 an hour).

THERAPIES FOR YOUR MIND

Mood and motivation are such important aspects of weight control that mental factors must always be considered alongside diet and fitness improvements.

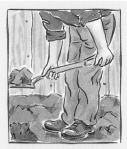

QUICK FITNESS TIP
Take an active interest in your garden. As well as burning energy, gardening can also help lift your mood.

Whether you need to strengthen your resolve or deal with the deeper emotional conflicts that underlie eating disorders, there are numerous therapies that work with the mind to assist in resolution of weight problems.

MEDITATION

The term "meditation" covers a wide range of practices, from simple prayer to the esoteric exercises of transcendental meditation. The principle aim of meditation is to bring the mind under control and to focus it in such a way that it becomes free of negative thoughts and emotions. Meditation is a therapeutically broad approach that is often incorporated in other techniques, including autogenics, hypnotherapy, behavioral psychology and psychotherapy. Most forms of meditation are carried out in a relatively passive state. Some, however, involve gentle movement or even quite vigorous physical activity, such as the dynamic meditation used by the Whirling Dervishes, a Muslim sect that achieves a trance state through spinning dances. A meditative element also forms an integral part of such oriental practices as yoga, t'ai chi, and qigong, in which breathing and rhythmical movement are used to harmonize body and mind.

Other Eastern-based systems of meditation use a mantra—a word chant or rhyme on which the individual focuses when meditating. Concentrating on a mantra helps to block out intrusive thoughts and calms the mind. A similar principle is used in the meditative technique of visualization.

Visualization

Mental imagery, or creative visualization, is a healthy way of ridding the body of negative images and stress and can be harnessed to produce a positive frame of mind. In a study carried out in the 1970s, U.S. cancer specialist Dr. Carl Simonton found that patients undergoing conventional cancer treatment had a better survival rate when they spent some time each day focusing on their bodies' healing processes at work, using mental images to which they could relate. Some might choose a military analogy, in which they imagined white blood cells as an army advancing on the tumor and overwhelming it. A young child might picture a team of dwarfs shoveling away the growth.

This method can be applied to many aspects of health, including weight problems. It doesn't have to be a biologically

HOW TO MEDITATE

Meditation is easy to do at home. Practicing every day, even for a short time, can be beneficial to a weight-control plan because it boosts positivity. Sitting comfortably with your back straight, breathe steadily and focus your mind on your breath as it flows in and out of your lungs. After a few minutes, visualize pleasant, tranquil surroundings such as the seashore or a woodland riverside. Playing a tape of soothing music can also help create the right mood.

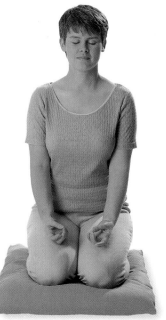

FINDING A POSITION
Adopt a comfortable position that allows you to breathe freely and deeply.

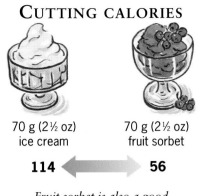

CUTTING CALORIES

70 g (2½ oz) ice cream

70 g (2½ oz) fruit sorbet

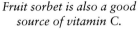

114 ⟷ **56**

Fruit sorbet is also a good source of vitamin C.

correct image. Just the process of regular visualization can initiate positive changes. For example, overweight individuals can picture fatty tissues dissolving and being carried out of the body. Or they may use visualization to create a goal for weight loss by seeing themselves exactly as they would like to be. They could also use the technique to discourage unhealthy eating by imagining what a tempting package of potato chips or chocolate bar will do to their bodies. Visualization is limited only by imagination.

HYPNOTHERAPY

The power of the mind can be harnessed for healing and self-development also through hypnotherapy. This approach may work better for individuals who find meditation and visualization difficult to sustain. In hypnotherapy an altered state of consciousness is induced by the practitioner, who then offers positive suggestions to the patient. For people who have weight problems these may center on understanding and overcoming addictive tendencies.

Hypnotherapy became popular with many psychologists in the 1800s, but then lost favor at the turn of the 20th century, as a means of getting faster results and a more accurate analysis of a patient's problems. While in the trance-like state induced by a hypnotherapist, a patient is open to suggestions from the practitioner and to the free expression of his or her own emotions.

When a therapist wishes to impart positive suggestions to a patient who needs to exercise dietary restraint, the removal of some mental resistance to these ideas can be a great advantage. It can also clear the way for a more relaxed discussion of emotional conflicts, which may underlie cravings, bingeing habits, or other eating disorders.

Contrary to popular belief hypnotherapy does not generally entail a loss of control over your own mind, merely a release of some of your emotional inhibitions.

Autosuggestion

The principle of reinforcing the motivation of the mind by repeating positive suggestions to oneself was first developed by Emile Coué. He encouraged patients to set aside times for mental concentration when they could repeat affirmations that were appropriate to their needs. His most famous phrase, a type of mantra, was: "Every day, in every way, I am getting better and better." Coué's objective was to stimulate the

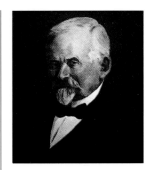

EMILE COUÉ
A French apothecary, Coué (1857–1926) became interested in autosuggestion when a patient's chronic illness was cured by a new medicine, which turned out to be just colored water. Now known as the placebo effect, this showed Coué how the mind has the ability to influence the physical condition of the body.

THE STATE OF HYPNOTIC TRANCE

The state of trance induced during a hynotherapy session is similar to that of daydreaming or sleepwalking. Therapists use this state to confront underlying emotional problems that may be causing physical symptoms in the patient.

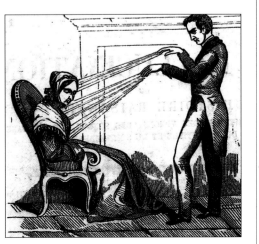

MESMERISM AND MODERN HYPNOTHERAPY
This picture, dating from about 1840, shows the "lines of force" that were believed to mesmerize a patient into a state of trance. Today, hypnosis is thought to work by inducing an altered state of highly relaxed consciousness during which the deepest recesses of the mind are made accessible.

GOALS FOR CHANGE

Cognitive behavior therapy can help motivate you toward your weight goals by prompting some positive changes.

▶ *A way of acting – to be more outgoing and confident about your self-image.*

▶ *A way of feeling – to be more positive.*

▶ *A way of thinking – to recognize and solve the underlying causes of your weight problem by employing positive thinking instead of negative thoughts.*

▶ *A way of coping – to take charge of your health and work toward improving your eating habits.*

patient's imagination and concentrate his or her mind. The principle could be applied equally well to the needs of a person with weight problems: "Every day, in every way, I am getting slimmer and trimmer."

Autogenic training is a modern variation of this. It uses techniques, which must be taught by an expert, that enable an individual to focus the mind in order to influence the body. These techniques include a series of basic exercises, such as imagining the arms growing heavy, coupled with a process of mental visualization of wellness.

BEHAVIORAL THERAPY

The capacity of the mind to learn new skills is the principle behind behavioral, or cognitive, therapy—a form of psychology based on a theory of learning. Certain patterns of behavior underlie various types of eating disorders, such as anorexia, bulimia, and bingeing habits. Just as you learn the essentials of social conduct throughout childhood by observing adults around you and receiving positive or negative reinforcements from them, so you can also be taught to change unwanted patterns of behavior that develop in adolescence or adulthood.

Certain situations give rise to nervous responses such as panic, fear, guilt, and depression. These reactions can be modified, thus enabling the patient to adapt to new stimuli or eradicate old problem traits of behavior. The origins of behavioral psychology lie in the experiments carried out by the Russian physiologist Ivan Pavlov (see

box, below), who trained dogs to associate the sound of a bell with the imminent arrival of their food until they eventually salivated in response to the bell alone, even when no food was forthcoming.

Cognitive behavioral therapy is one of the related forms of psychotherapy that is practiced today. It focuses mainly on a patient's present attitude rather than reaching back into his or her past. The aim of this form of therapy is to teach patients how to break out of negative thought patterns that may be underlying destructive forms of behavior and to begin to view themselves in a more positive light (see far left).

Overcoming weight-related anxieties

Whether you are underweight or overweight, eating too little or too much, or bingeing and vomiting (bulimia), there could be significant emotional factors responsible for your actions, so you may find it necessary to get professional guidance.

Behavioral psychotherapy can help with all types of eating disorders. For example, it can assist obese patients, through education about and reinforcement of healthy eating habits. With anorexic patients, a therapist usually concentrates on the root of the disease—a negative self-image. By helping a patient who suffers from bulimia to develop a habit of consuming healthy foods and to avoid bingeing, a therapist may succeed in reducing and eventually eradicating the guilt responses and negative feelings that cause the individual to vomit away calories.

Origins

Russian scientist Ivan Petrovich Pavlov discovered the conditioned reflex, which revealed the connection between external stimuli and physiological responses. His lifelong study was concentrated on the blood pressure, digestion, and nervous system of dogs. The ground-breaking research into the learned response of dogs showed how animals (and by implication, humans) can learn patterns of behavior that quickly become powerful and hard-to-change habits (such as bingeing, a characteristic of bulimia nervosa). His influence is still strong in modern-day behavioral psychology.

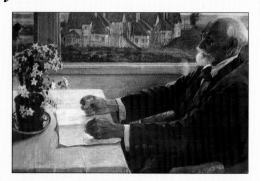

IVAN PAVLOV
Pavlov (1849-1936) pioneered research into learned bodily responses, for which he received a Nobel prize in 1904.

CHAPTER 7

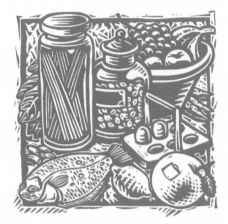

THE PROS AND CONS OF DIETS

Pressure to conform to the ideal slim physique, together with concerns over the negative health consequences of obesity, have led to an array of slimming techniques, books, programs, and aids that all promise rapid and successful weight loss. Many studies reveal that dieting is on the increase, with more than one-third of North American adults going on a weight-loss diet each year. In spite of these numbers, obesity is rising rapidly.

FACTS AND FALLACIES OF DIETING

Healthy eating habits are essential to avoid developing a bingeing and dieting pattern that is not only inefficient but can also lead to physical and emotional side effects.

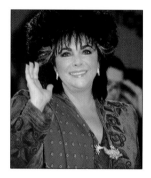

STAR'S STRUGGLE
Elizabeth Taylor's struggle to stay slim in order to conform to an idealized Hollywood film star image has resulted in a pattern of weight gain and dieting that is a classic example of yo-yo dieting.

All too often dieters turn to some sort of crash plan that promises fast results. In fact, North Americans spend some $25.3 billion each year on various fad diets. Experts believe that most of these plans are a waste of money and effort. People frequently find it so difficult to stick with the chosen regimen that they end up eating less than they should or they start bingeing. Perhaps it is necessary to question why new miracle diets are touted every year if the previous ones actually worked.

THE DIET INDUSTRY'S INFLUENCE
The highly lucrative diet industry tends to exploit the public's fears with myths about dieting that are not always backed by science. It also encourages the pursuit of unhealthy slenderness. Nutritionists advise that some diet plans are not only unsound but may also threaten health. In such cases the risk of the diet itself may outweigh those of being moderately overweight. Too many

diets work only in the short term, with weight being quickly regained when normal eating is resumed. If you are uncertain about the sensibleness of a diet plan, consult a registered dietitian, a qualified nutritionist, or your doctor.

DIETING AND YOUR BODY
Dieting, especially strict dieting, encourages you to disregard natural hunger signals from your body. This can have a severe effect on your metabolism and even cause emotional disturbances. For example, many people find that they develop an abnormal preoccupation with food, and this affects their social behavior and eating habits.

There is plenty of evidence that the body of anyone on a diet compensates by conserving energy, particularly during fasting or severe calorie restriction. The weight loss that occurs on a crash diet is short-lived because it is mainly water and protein from muscles (including the heart muscle) that

DIETS AND RELIGION

Many religions impose permanent or temporary dietary rules and recommendations on adherents. Roman Catholics, for example, might give up a favorite food during Lent. Fasting is also important in many faiths as a sign of reverence or self-discipline.

END OF RAMADAN
Moslems fast during Ramadan in the hope of having their sins pardoned. Even water is excluded during daylight hours. This picture shows the traditional prayer ceremony that marks the conclusion of the festival.

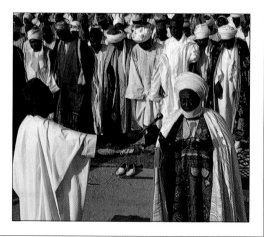

CAUTION
If you have a health problem you should consult your doctor before starting a diet of any kind. Pregnant women, children, and the elderly should seek guidance from a dietitian instead of dieting.

has been shed, rather than fat. It is extremely difficult to maintain a very low level of food intake over a long period of time, and most people find that they quickly return to their normal pattern of eating. In most cases, any weight lost is soon regained.

Risks of yo-yo dieting

Someone who is intent on losing weight can end up in a cycle of recurrent weight gains and losses known as yo-yo dieting. The weight lost is rarely maintained in the long term, frequent fluctuations in weight are common, and losing weight often becomes more difficult with each successive attempt.

Although it is clear that more and more people are riding this roller coaster of weight loss and gain, we don't know exactly why. We do know, however, that fat cells—once they are in place—never go away. They expand with weight gain and shrink when fat is drawn off for conversion to energy. One theory is that fat cells may emit a chemical plea for replenishment, thus beckoning people to eat more.

There can be serious health risks from yo-yo dieting. Among them are a loss of minerals from bones and irregularities in heart rate. Studies suggest that people whose weight is constantly fluctuating are at a 50 percent greater risk of developing heart disease.

The psychological damage of yo-yo dieting may be even greater than the physical consequences. Repeated cycles of weight loss and regain can contribute to a negative state of mind, including guilt feelings, as successful weight loss is followed by a sense of failure when the weight is regained. Chronic dieters are also more likely to feel insecure and have lower self-esteem than nondieters and are prone to eat more when anxious or depressed. This makes them more susceptible to unrealistic body images presented in the media and to the social and environmental influences that can lead to extremes in eating behavior.

Dieting has been implicated as the starting point for eating disorders such as anorexia nervosa and bulimia (see page 39). Both conditions sometimes begin with a simple attempt to lose weight. There are now many self-help organizations and clinics for those who find it hard to give up dieting and return to healthy eating patterns.

A SENSIBLE APPROACH

Crash dieting is not a solution. In fact, long-term weight loss and maintenance can be achieved only by making permanent changes to lifestyle and eating habits. A nutritionally balanced diet is essential for well-being and should not be compromised for weight goals. The good news is that current recommendations for healthy eating—a diet low in fat (particularly the saturated type) and high in fiber—can help anyone lose weight sensibly and permanently (see page 51 for what makes a healthy diet).

A healthful approach to eating not only helps you lose weight but also may prevent some serious health problems, such as the loss of bone minerals—which leads to osteoporosis—heart disease, intestinal disorders, and some types of cancer. Eating a wide variety of foods will provide all the nutrients essential for good health, and an increase in physical activity, which should always accompany a healthy eating plan, will help promote weight loss and well-being simultaneously.

BURNING OFF CALORIES: *Jogging*

Regular jogging can boost cardiovascular and respiratory systems, improve aerobic endurance, and tone and strengthen muscles. A jogging regimen should always be started gradually.

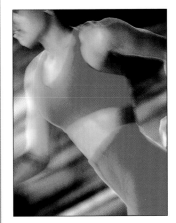

MUSCLE GROUPS BENEFITING
All leg muscles will benefit, but especially the thigh and calf muscles.

EQUIPMENT
Quality running shoes with arch supports and cushioned soles are vital to soften the impact. Thick socks help avoid blisters.

CALORIES BURNED
Jogging for 30 minutes at 11 km (7 miles) per hour will burn 360 calories (12 calories per minute).

DIETS FOR MEDICAL CONDITIONS

Many medical conditions can be improved by following special dietary guidelines; for those who have a weight problem as well, the diet must be planned with extra care.

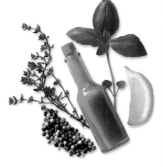

SALT ALTERNATIVES
Excess salt in the diet can aggravate hypertension. Healthier flavor enhancers include peppercorns, lemon juice, tabasco, and fresh herbs like thyme and basil.

With some disorders, following a strict dietary regimen can be a crucial factor in determining whether an individual suffers serious physical symptoms or remains fit and well.

DIABETES MELLITUS
This condition affects more than 10.5 million people in North America, although many more cases go undiagnosed. Dietary needs vary, depending on the type of diabetes and whether or not the individual is overweight. However, all diabetics need to follow a diet that is high in complex carbohydrates and low in simple sugars. This helps to prevent fluctuations in blood glucose levels, which result in hypoglycemia (low blood sugar) or hyperglycemia (high blood sugar). A high fiber intake also slows down the rate of absorption of glucose into the bloodstream and helps maintain normal glucose levels. Limiting saturated fat is also recommended, to prevent the cardiovascular problems that are common in people with diabetes.

HIGH CHOLESTEROL
Individuals with high blood cholesterol, or hypercholesterolemia, can lower lipid levels by as much as 14 percent if they adhere to a diet that is low in saturated fats. Meat and whole-milk dairy products contain high levels of saturated fatty acids. People with severe hypercholesterolemia may also need to take cholesterol-lowering drugs to reduce

SYMPTOMS OF DIABETES MELLITUS

Diabetes is a chronic disease in which the body either does not produce or does not fully utilize insulin and thus cannot properly metabolize carbohydrates and, to a lesser extent, protein and fat. Glucose builds up in the blood, and the kidneys begin to excrete the excess in the urine. There are two major forms—insulin-dependent, which requires daily injections of insulin and a special diet and exercise regimen, and non-insulin-dependent, which often can be controlled by diet and exercise alone. The second type usually develops later in life and is most common among overweight people.

TAKING ACTION
Diabetes is a serious disease. If you experience any of the signs shown here, consult your doctor right away.

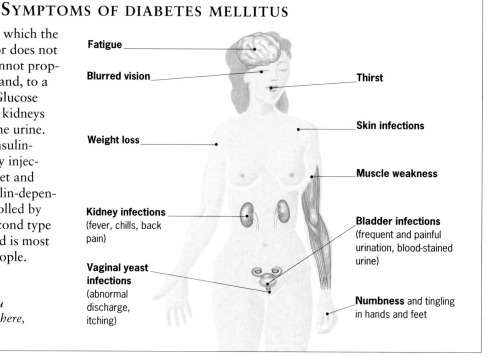

Fatigue

Blurred vision

Thirst

Skin infections

Weight loss

Muscle weakness

Kidney infections (fever, chills, back pain)

Bladder infections (frequent and painful urination, blood-stained urine)

Vaginal yeast infections (abnormal discharge, itching)

Numbness and tingling in hands and feet

CUTTING CHOLESTEROL

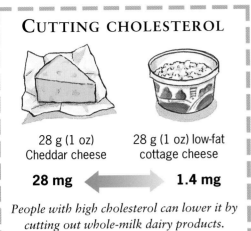

28 g (1 oz) Cheddar cheese	28 g (1 oz) low-fat cottage cheese
28 mg ⬅️➡️	**1.4 mg**

People with high cholesterol can lower it by cutting out whole-milk dairy products.

the risk of cardiovascular disease. Increasing their intake of soluble fiber—found in oats, legumes, fruits, and root vegetables—can help lower levels of cholesterol by preventing its absorption by the body.

HIGH BLOOD PRESSURE
Cutting down on saturated fat is important, too, for reducing high blood pressure, or hypertension. Certain people at risk for hypertension can benefit also from reducing the salt (sodium) in their diet. Current advice recommends keeping sodium intake to between 2,200 and 3,300 milligrams per day (the equivalent of 1 to 1½ teaspoons of salt), particularly for people who are salt sensitive. Eating plenty of vegetables and fruits that are high in potassium—bananas, citrus fruits, avocados, beans, and whole-grain products, for instance—can help, since potassium counteracts excess sodium.

CELIAC DISEASE
Special diets that totally exclude the protein gluten are essential for people who have celiac disease. This condition, caused by a sensitivity to gluten, is a hereditary defect that usually shows up at an early age. In those affected, gluten damages the lining of the small intestine, leading to impaired absorption of nutrients. Symptoms can include diarrhea, bloating, weight loss, and anemia. Scrupulously avoiding foods that contain gluten can quickly reverse the symptoms. Gluten is present in wheat, rye, and to a lesser extent barley and oats, and all processed foods that contain any of these cereals, so it is necessary to read food labels scrupulously. Alternative sources of energy and nutrients include beans, rice, potatoes,

corn, and nuts. Gluten-free bread and other cereals are also available from health food stores. A dietitian can help plan a balanced diet that includes all the vital nutrients in the required amounts. She may also advise taking a vitamin and mineral supplement.

FOOD ALLERGY/INTOLERANCE
People suffering from food intolerance or allergy will improve once they exclude the problem foods from their diets. Symptoms of food allergy or intolerance often include excessive tiredness, diarrhea, migraine, and even potentially fatal reactions such as anaphylactic shock. Common culprits include milk, eggs, fish, shellfish, nuts, soy beans, and some food additives. Often it is difficult to pinpoint the exact cause, and an elimination diet may be necessary. This involves excluding all but a few known safe foods from the diet and then gradually reintroducing other foods to see which ones cause a reaction. This approach requires patience and willpower to succeed. The advice of a doctor or dietitian is also essential to avoid the potential health risks of a restricted diet.

KIDNEY COMPLAINTS
People who have kidney problems need to follow a low-protein diet to prevent further damage to their kidneys. Sodium, potassium, and fluids may also be restricted, depending on the condition and extent of kidney damage. These diets require professional advice from a dietitian and plenty of motivation and perseverance on the part of the patient, as they are very difficult to follow.

CYSTIC FIBROSIS
People with cystic fibrosis are advised to follow a high-energy, high-protein diet. This hereditary condition, caused by defective genes inherited from both parents, is characterized by an overproduction of mucus in the lungs and pancreas. Food is not properly digested before passing into the large bowel, causing diarrhea and deficiencies in the fat-soluble vitamins A, D, E, and K. Apart from taking pancreatic enzymes in capsule form to aid digestion, a diet high in energy, particularly in the form of fat, is essential to meet nutritional demands. The need to maintain adequate nutrient levels and prevent weight loss far outweighs any increased risk of cardiovascular disease from following a high-fat diet.

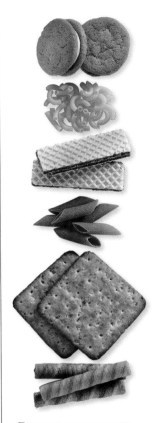

GLUTEN-FREE FOODS
People with celiac disease, who cannot eat cereal-based products containing gluten, need not miss out on tasty treats. Gluten-free cookies and savory snacks are available from larger pharmacies, some supermarkets, and most health food stores.

CHOOSING A DIET

To be useful, a diet should promote steady, gradual weight loss and a long-term change to healthy eating habits. It is essential to look beyond the hype and judge a diet's merits for yourself.

Low-fat foods that fill you up

Complex carbohydrates like potatoes, bread, pasta, and cereal, which form the major part of any balanced diet, are essentially low-fat foods. It is the toppings and spreads eaten with them—butter and cheese on a baked potato, a creamy sauce on pasta, whole milk on cereal—that raise the fat content and calorie count. Choose low-fat options such as nonfat yogurt or sour cream for potatoes, tomato-based sauces for pasta, and skim or low-fat milk for cereal.

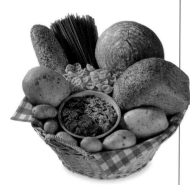

FIBER PROVIDERS
Fiber, essential to health (see pages 60–61), can be found in whole-grain breads, cereals, and pasta, also potato skins and brown rice.

Despite the sound dietary guidelines offered by the U.S. Department of Agriculture, Health Canada, and trained dietitians to help individuals with special dietary needs, the majority of people who want to lose weight prefer to follow a published diet. This section examines some of the most popular diets of recent years.

AVOIDING SEVERITY

Most diets can be safely followed for a short period of time or adapted to avoid health risks. Some, however, have little or no scientific basis and call for such extreme measures, they can be dangerous to your health.

Fasting

This involves giving up food altogether to achieve rapid weight loss and drinking lots of water during the process. It is sometimes claimed, without scientific proof, that toxins will be flushed out of the body and thus health will be improved. But totally depriving your body of food for any length of time is dangerous, and in susceptible individuals it can lead to an attack of gout, lowered blood pressure, even heart failure. Often the weight lost is rapidly regained, once normal eating resumes. Children, pregnant women, and the elderly should never attempt fasting.

Rotation diet

In this approach total daily calorie intakes are alternated from week to week to avoid the metabolic rate decreases believed to occur when a low-calorie diet is followed for a long time. Initially 600 calories a day are allowed, followed by 900, and then 1,200; the cycle is repeated until the desired weight is achieved. There is no scientific evidence that the body's metabolism can be tricked in this way and, at 600 calories a day, it may not be possible to obtain all the vitamins and minerals that are needed.

Mono diets

The basis of such diets is one food, which is allowed in unlimited amounts to the virtual exclusion of everything else. These "wonder" foods are supposed to contain substances that enhance the fat-burning process and speed weight loss. Fruits such as papaya and pineapple have been cited, but while it is true they contain enzymes that can break up proteins, there is no evidence that they aid the digestive system in any way. There is no magic involved. Such a restricted food choice makes it very hard to consume a lot of calories, so some weight loss is inevitable, particularly if the food is low in calories. These diets are not recommended, as they are far too low in energy, and no single food can provide all the necessary nutrients.

Scarsdale diet

Plenty of protein, in the form of poultry, fish, and eggs, is the mainstay of this diet. Fats and carbohydrates are limited. Since there is no restriction on any lean protein food, the plan provides about 43 percent of calories from protein, while the current recommendation suggests 10 to 15 percent as adequate. It is suggested that this diet not be followed for longer than 14 days. Unfortunately, few people, can resolve their weight problems this quickly.

Low-carbohydrate diet

This plan aims to restrict intake of carbohydrate-rich foods such as bread, pasta, and rice. The principle behind it is that when starchy foods are cut from the diet, energy intake is automatically reduced. However, the fat intake tends to be high, which goes against current recommendations for reducing the risk of heart disease. The danger in this diet is that it upsets the basic metabolism and deprives the brain of glucose, causing dizziness and other complications.

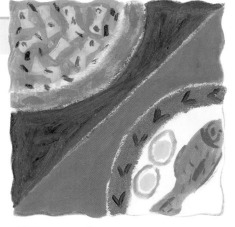

THE HAY DIET

The theory that proteins and carbohydrates should not be mixed in the same meal was made popular by Dr. William Hay in the early 1900s. He believed that conditions such as indigestion, allergies, and skin disorders were due to an accumulation of toxins in the body caused by eating too much meat and too many processed foods. He recommended that vegetables and fruits form the bulk of a diet, while concentrated sources of proteins, carbohydrates, and fats be consumed sparingly. Carbohydrate foods such as potatoes and pasta should not be eaten in the same meal as protein foods like meat and dairy products. Meals should be at least four hours apart to allow digestion.

 ### Rationale
The theory of this diet is that for digestion carbohydrates need an alkaline environment while proteins require acidic conditions. Mixing the two is said to neutralize the medium and cause malabsorption and inadequate digestion. Scientists today discredit this theory; many foods contain both carbohydrates and proteins and the digestive system handles both simultaneously.

 ### Risks
This diet perpetuates the myth that certain foods can be combined to help a person lose weight. One unforeseen effect is that some people follow the Hay diet principles by cutting back too much on carbohydrates. As a result, the proportion of fat in the diet may increase inadvertently, possibly leading to weight gain and health problems such as coronary heart disease.

Benefits
Despite problems with the Hay diet's rationale, weight loss can be achieved by following this approach because of the reduction in fat and calories that results from restricting the range of foods allowed. The diet also encourages a healthy consumption of fruits and vegetables and a reduction in fat intake, which is in line with what nutritionists today recommend.

VERY-LOW-CALORIE DIET

This diet became very popular in the early 1980s as a means of rapid weight loss. It is usually based around a flavored milkshake or snack bar that supplies the recommended daily amounts of vitamins, proteins, minerals, and fat in up to 600 calories. Although satisfactory for short-term use (a few days), any weight lost is likely to be regained when normal eating habits are resumed. This diet is too severe for a long-term program of weight control and does nothing to encourage healthy eating habits, which is essential if weight loss is to be maintained.

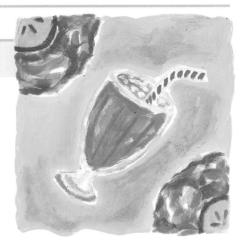

 ### Rationale
This diet depends on the fact that if the body is given a low-energy intake it is compelled to draw the additional energy it needs from fat stores: rapid weight loss will be inevitable. The problem is that the body becomes efficient at functioning on less energy, so the metabolic rate declines, and the body tends to use up lean tissue from muscles—including the heart—as well as fat.

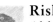 ### Risks
Although temporary use of this diet is unlikely to cause harm, in the long term it may present a risk to health, especially since most people quickly regain the weight lost and some of them may embark on the yo-yo syndrome. A limit of four weeks is advised. Pregnant women, people who have chronic health problems, children, and the elderly should never follow these plans.

Benefits
These very-low-calorie meals are usually complete in vitamins and minerals, whereas home cooked meals often are not. A more acceptable way of using such a diet is as a replacement for just one or two of the smaller meals of the day, continuing with the normal main meal. In this way a calorie intake of about 1,000 per day can be achieved with little danger to health.

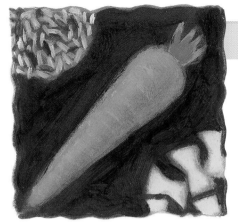

LOW-FAT DIET

A diet that is based on significantly lowering total fat intake—by excluding or limiting items that are particularly rich in fat such as fried foods, many types of meat, whole-milk dairy products, and oily salad dressings—can be considered a low-fat diet. Usually a higher intake of starchy foods, fruits, and vegetables is suggested to bring the diet more in line with healthy eating recommendations. Weight loss is usually successful on this diet and is likely to be maintained, provided that the low-fat eating principles are adopted on a permanent basis.

 ### Rationale
The principle behind this diet is similar to that of the low-carbohydrate diet (see page 104), in that avoidance of certain foods will lead to a reduction in total calories. This diet makes sense, because fat is the most concentrated source of energy, providing twice as many calories per gram as carbohydrate or protein. It is also the least satiating, making it easy to overconsume.

 ### Risks
Some proponents of low-fat diets make misleading claims, such as perpetuating the myth that cellulite is caused by toxic substances and that these diets can help spot-reduce fat. Also, such plans can mistakenly put too much emphasis on reducing only total fat intake, when, in fact, the most important goal should be to reduce saturated fats from animal foods.

Benefits
Currently, people tend to eat more fat than they need, and low-fat diets can be helpful in bringing fat intake down to recommended levels. Reducing saturated fat in the diet has proven to reduce risks of heart disease. The other advantage is that this approach is easy to maintain. Starchy foods add bulk to the diet and are more filling. Eating habits may also change for the better.

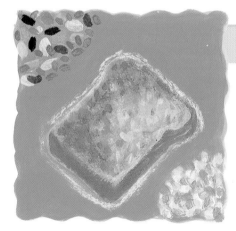

HIGH-FIBER DIET

This diet includes a high intake of fiber from sources such as vegetables, fruits, whole-grain cereals, and nuts. Provided this means a reduction in daily calorie intake, a high-fiber diet can result in weight loss. It is important to choose a balanced range of foods to ensure that the body receives all the vitamins, minerals, and other nutrients essential for good health. Fiber intake should not exceed 35 g per day, because intake above this level can interfere with the body's mineral supply. Remember that there is a difference between soluble and insoluble fiber (see below, left) and you need both for a balanced diet. Fiber should be increased gradually to avoid gasiness and bloating.

Rationale
A high-fiber regimen can aid weight loss by increasing bulk in the diet, quickly providing a sensation of fullness on fewer calories. This principle forms the basis of many popular diets. Fiber is vital to health. Insoluble fiber (in rice, bran, and nuts) aids digestion and is highly satiating, while soluble fiber (in bread, beans, fruits, and vegetables) can help lower cholesterol.

 ### Risks
The amount of fiber usually recommended is very high and may produce side effects such as flatulence and diarrhea. People with irritable bowel syndrome, or IBS, may also find that their condition is exacerbated. A very large intake of bran can bind minerals such as iron and zinc and prevent their absorption by the body, although soluble fiber can increase their absorption.

Benefits
Most nutritionists agree that a high-fiber intake is beneficial, especially in the form of cereals, legumes, vegetables, and fruits rather than pills. It can help reduce the risk of some kinds of cancer, particularly cancer of the colon, and also helps prevent other gut problems like diverticulosis. The decrease in fat that often accompanies this diet is a bonus.

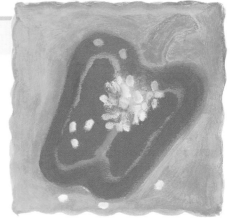

VEGETARIAN DIET

This diet excludes all animal flesh and products. A vegan diet also excludes animal by-products such as milk and other dairy items and eggs. Vegetarians who rely heavily on dairy products must take care to choose low-fat varieties. Cutting out meat is helpful for reducing saturated fats and cholesterol, but meat is an important source of high quality (complete) protein, iron, and vitamin B_{12}. The complete protein must be replaced by combining complementary plants—legumes (vegetables that bear seed pods) with grains, seeds, or nuts. It may also be necessary to take a vitamin or mineral supplement.

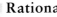 ### Rationale
The theory of vegetarianism when practiced for healthy eating is that the low amount of fat and animal protein consumed will be easier for the digestion, aid liver functioning, and detoxify the body. Because the diet is high in fruit and vegetables, which are low in calories, weight loss is usually possible, but it is also important to keep a check on fat for a lower total calorie intake.

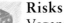 ### Risks
Vegans should eat foods fortified with vitamin B_{12}, as this is found naturally only in animal products. Another area of concern for vegetarians is not getting enough iron and zinc and sometimes calcium from their diets. They must also combine complementary plant proteins—such as rice with lentils, bread with peanut butter, pasta with peas—to obtain complete protein.

Benefits
A well-planned vegetarian diet is healthful. An emphasis on whole-grain cereals, beans, brown rice, fruits, and vegetables will ensure a good intake of fiber, iron, and the B vitamins (except B_{12}). The exclusion of meat and, for vegans, dairy products, dramatically reduces saturated fat in the diet, thus lowering the risk of many disorders, including heart disease.

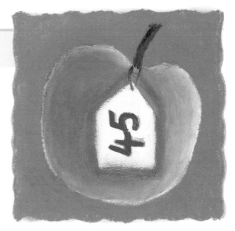

CALORIE-COUNTED DIET

This diet involves weighing and assessing the calorie content of food items in order to regulate intake of total calories at a level low enough to produce weight loss. It can be extremely difficult to weigh food accurately and mistakes can be made in calculating total calorie intake. Frequently, people stop weighing food after a few days, and over time their portion sizes increase, calorie intakes creep up, and the rate of weight loss declines. Some people can also become unduly preoccupied with calorie counting, losing sight of equally important nutritional considerations like fat content.

Rationale
This diet limits energy intake through strict control of calories. Thus, all types of foods are permitted, provided a certain calorie limit is not exceeded. If this limit is below the energy requirements of the individual, weight will be lost. Almost all diets are based on some form of energy restriction, although many come disguised as magic formulas and make false nutritional claims.

 ### Risks
Calorie-counting diets that omit some food groups while emphasizing others, and those that do not properly balance nutrient intake should be avoided. These can be tailored to better standards, but some dieters may lack the nutritional knowledge to make adequate choices. When allowed to select their own foods by counting calories, some people make less healthful choices.

Benefits
This type of diet is popular because it does not require any food restrictions and can be adapted to suit individual needs and taste. The plan can promote good eating habits through education, when people learn how foods vary in their calorie contents and how to tailor food shopping toward low-calorie options. Fat content should be monitored as well as calories.

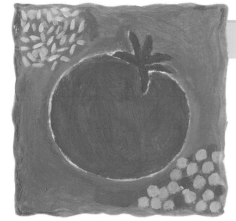

THE PRITIKIN DIET

Developed in the 1970s by Nathan Pritikin, this diet characteristically is high in unrefined, complex carbohydrate foods, primarily whole grains, fruits, and vegetables, and very low in meat and animal by-products (and protein in general), caffeine, fat, cholesterol, sugar, and salt. Nathan Pritikin was an engineer and inventor, who during the Second World War designed and manufactured army munitions. After developing heart problems he became interested in diet and health and created a program to re-educate people about healthy eating, in order to combat the threat of heart disease.

 ### Rationale
Pritikin's approach combines diet and exercise regimens designed to promote fitness, reduce weight, and lengthen life. He believed that a drastic reduction in fat (to less than 10 percent of total calories) and severe restrictions in sugar, caffeine, cholesterol, salt, and alcohol should have beneficial effects on the body and significantly reduce the risk of heart disease.

 ### Risks
The bulk of the Pritikin diet is derived from vegetables, so protein and fat intake are usually below the recommended daily amounts. The rigidity of the diet makes it difficult to stick to and therefore unlikely to change people's eating habits, which is vital for long-term weight maintenance. Cutting out all dairy products also limits the amount of calcium in the diet.

 ### Benefits
The Pritikin diet includes a lot of sound advice and particularly stresses the link between diet and exercise. The programs have shown good results for clients in Pritikin's Longevity Center in California, where significant improvements in blood cholesterol have been documented. But similar improvements can be achieved by following less restrictive diets.

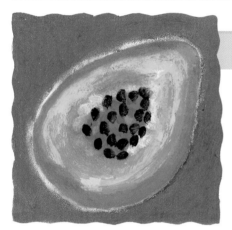

THE RAW-ENERGY DIET

Foods that are processed or cooked in any way are excluded from this diet, and between 50 and 75 percent of total calorie intake is from raw fruits, vegetables, nuts, and seeds. An inventive array of salads and fruit desserts are recommended as well as no-cook soups, home-made yogurt, nut loaves, and unbaked cakes. The diet considerably lowers fat intake and calorie counts and therefore results in weight loss. However, it can be difficult and time consuming to prepare all meals from raw ingredients. Some of the ideas could be incorporated into less complicated healthful eating plans.

Rationale
Many people claim that a diet high in raw food helps to improve vitality, detoxify the body, and assist weight loss. The diet is thought to be particularly beneficial to those with such conditions as arthritis and diabetes. There are claims that live enzymes contained in raw foods help the body to boost its immune system and fight disease, but these are as yet unproven.

 ### Risks
This diet may be deficient in some nutrients such as iron and vitamin B_{12}, which are abundant in animal foods. Taken to extremes over a long period, the diet may also lead to other nutritional deficiencies. If too little fat is eaten, absorption of the fat soluble vitamins may be inadequate. The diet is unsuitable for children, pregnant women, and the elderly.

Benefits
Eating mostly vegetables and fruits does provide the body with plenty of fiber and many nutrients, particularly potassium and vitamins A and C and other antioxidants that may help prevent cancer. The raw-food diet has a low-energy density, which can be useful for a weight loss plan because it helps suppress appetite and fills you up without taking in too many calories.

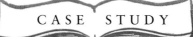
The Yo-yo Dieter

Yo-yo dieters repeatedly try to achieve an ideal weight by dieting. Typically, they spend several months of each year following a weight-reducing plan, with periods of normal eating in between. Unfortunately, many people find that they quickly regain weight when they come off a diet, and so they follow a continuous cycle of weight loss and weight gain.

Alison is a 26-year-old hairdresser who recently married. She has never been slim and has always had a sweet tooth. She dieted in preparation for her wedding to David and lost 15 kg (33 lb), reaching 60 kg (132 lb), a healthy weight for her height. Married life suited Alison, and her eating habits became very relaxed again. After six months she was back to her original weight, but as her vacation approached she decided to diet again and lost 10 kg (22 lb). On her return, her weight crept up once more and she soon weighed 70 kg (154 lb). Alison realizes that this pattern of weight fluctuation is likely to continue throughout her life unless she makes permanent changes.

WHAT SHOULD ALISON DO?

Alison should start by keeping a food diary of everything she eats for at least two weeks. A diary often helps highlight where a person is going wrong, and can be useful when discussing the problem with a partner or health professional. She should also identify ways of improving her diet. For instance, she must avoid skipping lunch, because she then eats a chocolate bar or cookies in the afternoon to keep herself going. A low-calorie sandwich would have less effect on her weight and be more beneficial to her health. It is also important for Alison to think about a long-term exercise program, as this will help increase her energy expenditure and overall fitness.

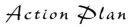

Action Plan

FITNESS
Begin a regular exercise program to help keep weight down and provide a distraction from eating snacks and sweets.

EATING HABITS
Eat lunch every day, preferably something high in protein and fiber—for example, a sandwich of turkey on whole-wheat bread or a baked potato topped with low-fat cheese and broccoli. Substitute fruit for high-fat snacks.

FAMILY
Talk to David about the need for support and ask if he will join her in some form of exercise.

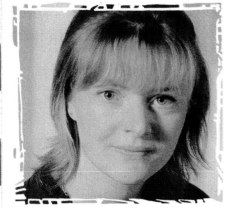

FITNESS
Lack of exercise makes it difficult to reduce or stabilize weight.

EATING HABITS
Irregular eating habits can lead to snacking on high-fat or sugary foods.

FAMILY
A partner can play an important role in offering practical and emotional support to someone who is trying to regulate her weight.

HOW THINGS TURNED OUT FOR ALISON

Alison now carefully structures her daily meals and snacks only on healthful, low-calorie foods. She bicycles 7 km (4 miles) to work every day and her fitness has increased dramatically, helping her to lose 7 kg (15 lb). She has given up chocolate, apart from the occasional treat, and always eats a substantial lunch, usually brown-bagging it from home. She does not think she will ever be thin, but is happy that her weight is stable and within a healthy range for her height.

DIET AIDS AND GIMMICKS

The so-called weight-loss aids available today range from special foods to pills, creams, and patches. Unfortunately, few of these items seem to be of genuine value.

Health food stores, diet clinics, and even supermarkets now offer aids to quick slimming. It can be difficult to know, however, if any of these things are going to be useful. Some, when used as directed, can help jump-start a diet, but most are of very little value and a few can even be dangerous. The important point to keep in mind is that there are no magic solutions to weight loss.

DIET BOOKS

For many people, purchase of a diet book is the first step in their weight-loss project. Often they turn to new diets because old ones have failed. New diet books are always appearing, but few deliver an entirely new concept. Diets work only if they restrict calorie intake relative to energy expenditure, although from a nutritional point of view some are clearly better than others. Diet plans that don't give helpful advice on who needs to lose weight, or that encourage rapid weight loss or allow only a limited selection of foods should be avoided.

A good diet book can be a real help, however, in terms of both practical advice and inspiration. It should assist you in establishing whether or not you actually need to lose weight and advise a regimen in line with healthful dietary recommendations. Severe food restrictions are unnecessary, and you should aim for a weight loss of 0.5 to 1 kg (1 to 2 lb) a week.

SPECIAL DIET FOODS

Meal replacements (see left) are becoming increasingly popular, along with other low-calorie foods and slimming aids. These products can be high in sugar, however, and if they work, it is only because total calorie intake is dramatically restricted. Advertisements for meal replacement plans usually make claims for rapid weight loss, but these diets do nothing to change eating habits. This means that as soon as you resume your normal diet, any weight you lost is likely to be regained. Therefore, they are unsuitable for long-term use. Another drawback is cost. It is generally cheaper to reduce your food intake than to buy meal replacements.

Supplements

Many health food stores sell herbal supplements, which their manufacturers claim promote fast, effective weight loss. These

---

MEAL REPLACEMENTS

Meal replacements, usually in the form of bars or milk-shakes, are meant to replace breakfast, lunch, or both, while providing all the nutrients essential to health but with fewer calories. No laws exist to control their nutritional quality, however, and some products don't provide enough protein and fiber. People who use meal replacements often find that they at least help them get used to eating less. These products have increased dramatically in popularity since 1990.

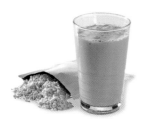

A MEAL IN A SHAKE
Although meal replacements can be useful in a calorie-controlled diet, they are only a short-term solution and do nothing to encourage healthy eating habits.

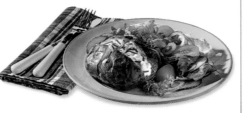

REAL FOOD ALTERNATIVES
The calorie content of a light meal, such as this baked potato with cottage cheese and a salad, is about the same as a meal replacement but more filling and satisfying.

usually contain various plant substances such as lecithin, kelp, ginseng, or ginger. Their ability to assist in weight loss has never been proven scientifically. However, studies done with evening primrose, a native wildflower that grows from Newfoundland to British Columbia and south to Florida, have shown some promise that it might aid weight loss, especially among persons with a family history of obesity.

There are other substances touted as having the ability to burn fat, and they are sold at inflated prices. One of these is chromium picolinate, an easily digested form of chromium, which acts in conjunction with insulin to burn glucose—the body's major fuel. Many claims have been made for this mineral, the most notable being that it helps build muscle, melts away fat, and boosts energy. So far, these effects have not been substantiated in scientific experiments.

GIMMICKS

The diet industry is constantly devising new slimming aids. Some are gadgets: special clothing that its marketers claim can increase your metabolic rate, and massage machines and electric pads that are supposed to exercise your muscles by contracting them. Other gimmicks such as diet creams and body wraps are popular even though there is no evidence proving their efficacy in the long run. Some, such as weight-loss patches, can even be dangerous.

Diet creams

These have been invented to target cellulite, despite the fact that experts insist cellulite is just normal fat. It is suggested that fat cells beneath the skin disintegrate when the cream is rubbed onto the targeted area,

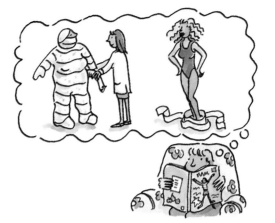

although scientific evidence does not support this claim. These creams may contain substances that cause a local increase in blood flow, which in turn makes the skin tighten slightly, thus improving its look. However, these creams do not reduce the amount of fat present, and even the slight firmness of the skin that occurs with the massaging action is short-term and will disappear when you stop using the cream.

Body wraps—the easy way out?

Body wraps have become fashionable at many health spas and clinics as an easy way to lose some weight. This usually entails being covered with mud and then wrapped in bandages. The theory is to open up the pores of the skin and draw out the toxins from the fat beneath. In fact, any reduction in weight is due to water loss through sweating and is quickly replenished by drinking fluids. The idea that some fat deposition is due to toxins has no scientific basis.

Weight-loss patches

Weight-loss patches promise to increase your metabolism by passing substances such as iodine into the bloodstream. Iodine is a mineral needed by the body to make thyroid hormone and is essential for controlling the rate of metabolism. Although one's metabolic rate does decrease if iodine is deficient in the diet, it cannot be increased by taking extra iodine. In any case, iodine deficiency is very rare. The amount of iodine present in skin patches is usually too small to have any effect. Thyroid hormone preparations do increase the metabolic rate, but in people with normal thyroid function they have a range of adverse effects, including loss of muscle tissue and heart problems, and are not suitable as an aid to weight loss.

HOLD ON TO REALITY!
Treatments such as body wraps cannot perform miracles. Reaching an ideal body weight is a long-term commitment, and there really is no substitute for eating healthily and increasing physical activity. However, you can use special treatments to reward yourself for successful weight loss.

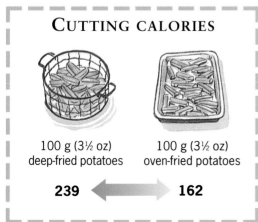

CUTTING CALORIES

100 g (3½ oz) deep-fried potatoes

100 g (3½ oz) oven-fried potatoes

239 ← → **162**

DIET PILLS

The race to find a magic way to dissolve fat effortlessly has prompted development of "miracle pills." At best they are harmless, containing herbal ingredients or vitamins that have no effect; at worst they can cause side effects such as nausea, high blood pressure, insomnia, and even hallucinations.

New diet pills are advertised in the press all the time, some claiming breakthrough scientific discoveries. Most of these claims are unsubstantiated by scientific proof.

There are various drugs and natural products used to treat obesity, and they work in different ways. For example, diuretics remove water from the body by prompting urination, thus weight loss is fast but this is water, not fat, and is quickly regained. Caffeine and certain herbal mixtures also act as diuretics. Bulking agents in some diet pills claim to make you feel full more quickly if you take them just before meals. These include natural forms of fiber such as guar gum and sugar beet fiber. If taken in large amounts they can cause intestinal blockages, but most products contain amounts too small to create this problem.

Many over-the-counter preparations used to treat asthma or hay fever contain theophylline and ephedrine—two drugs that are known to increase the metabolic rate. Theophylline is related to caffeine and is present in various plants such as tea, coffee, cocoa, and the cola plant. Ephedrine is also a naturally occurring drug that has been used in China for at least 5,000 years under the name of ma huang. However, clinical trials to assess its effectiveness in the treatment of obesity are lacking. Misuse of these products has been linked to heart attacks and even deaths. Dosage instructions and precautions should be followed and only government approved products should be used.

Prescription drugs

A number of prescription drugs can assist in weight loss. Some, such as amphetamines and related compounds, are potentially addictive and have possible side effects that include nervousness, high blood pressure, palpitations, headaches, dizziness, insomnia, dry mouth, tremor, itching, and rashes. There has been concern within the health industry that some diet clinics may be too quick to dispense these drugs, sometimes even to people who already have a healthy

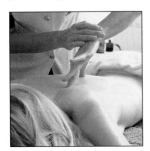

TREAT YOURSELF
Massage can improve the circulation, helping to tone skin and muscle, but it cannot actually produce weight loss. Its main benefit lies in relaxing the body and enhancing general mental well-being, essential for a healthy lifestyle and maintaining the motivation needed for dieting.

> ### CAUTION
> *Diuretics should be avoided, except when prescribed for hypertension. They can disturb the body's fluid balance by removing too much potassium along with water, and lead to dehydration, especially in diabetic patients. Blood sugar levels are also adversely affected.*

body weight. It is unwise to attend a diet clinic or take any drugs or diet pills without checking first with your family doctor.

A limited number of drugs are available on prescription to obese people for losing weight; all carry a risk of dependency and so cannot be prescribed for more than 12 weeks as a rule. Some work by increasing serotonin levels in the brain, helping to curb appetite and elevate mood. These are not miracle cures, but they are relatively safe when used as prescribed and in conjunction with a sensible eating plan. Clinical trials show that weight is often regained when treatment is stopped.

The pharmaceutical industry is always searching for new drugs to treat obesity. Increasingly, though, it is recognized that there is unlikely to be a miracle cure that promotes weight loss without effort. Drugs can help reinforce and maximize weight loss achieved by changes in diet and lifestyle.

SPOT REDUCTION

Many popular diets provide detailed advice on how to slim down parts of the body, particularly the hips and thighs. This is, unfortunately, another myth: it is not possible to spot reduce fat except by liposuction, a surgical technique that removes fat from beneath the skin by aspirating it through a needle. Liposuction can have unpleasant side effects and leave permanent scars, and some studies suggest that the fat removed may be quickly replaced.

Body shape and fat deposition are mostly determined genetically, and weight loss cannot be targeted to a particular part of the body. When you go on a diet fat is lost first from the abdominal cavity, shoulders, and face, and then the hips and thighs. Exercise, however, can alter body shape by improving muscle tone, and should be an integral part of any weight-loss plan.

JOINING A WEIGHT-LOSS GROUP

Diet groups have helped millions of overweight people lose weight successfully. Many experts agree that they offer some of the best techniques to help you lose weight and keep it off.

Diet books and individual weight-loss programs, as useful as they are, lack the help and support that comes through contact with other people who are going through a similar process. Dieters who join groups are also exposed to role models who have managed to lose weight and keep it off by changing their lifestyles.

CHOOSING A GROUP

There are many weight-loss groups from which to choose. Some may be listed in your telephone directory, or your doctor may be able to suggest a good one. Diet groups are not for everyone, and the best way to find out if a particular one suits you is to attend a couple of meetings and see for yourself. Large commercial diet clubs such as Weight Watchers and Jenny Craig are among the best-known in the business, but there are also plenty of nonprofit community groups to choose from, some run by dietitians.

Commercial clubs usually charge a fee to join and then weekly meeting fees after that. For your money, you receive a diet and exercise plan, a private weigh-in each week, and group talks on how to improve eating habits. Personal attention is available for those who need it. Diet plans can vary, but many clubs offer sound nutritional advice with an emphasis on low-fat, high-carbohydrate diets. Another positive aspect is that they do not encourage rapid weight loss. A study published in 1990, which tested the efficacy of various diets in overweight individuals, found the methods of weight-control clubs to be among the most successful

continued on page 116

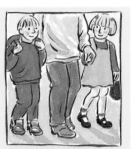

QUICK FITNESS TIP
Try to avoid taking unnecessary trips in the car. Instead, walk whenever possible, such as when taking the children to school or shopping locally.

LIFE ON A HEALTH FARM

Health farms, spas, and weekend clinics provide luxurious surroundings where people can detoxify or lose weight. Guests are removed from the distractions of everyday life and are encouraged to exercise, eat sensibly, and relax.

Services such as massage, exercise classes, saunas, hydrotherapy, dietary advice, lectures, beauty therapy, reflexology, osteopathy, and aromatherapy are usually available, together with sport and leisure activities like riding or golf.

Guests may have a medical consultation to work out a personal program, and by the time they leave they will have learned about and experienced lifestyle changes they can adopt permanently.

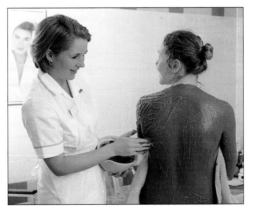

BEAUTY IS SKIN DEEP
Seaweed beauty treatments cleanse the skin, enhance the body's appearance, and lull the recipient into a relaxed state of mind.

Weight-loss Club Leader

For people who are concerned about being overweight but find it hard to stick to a diet, the informal, supportive environment of a weight-loss club can offer the encouragement they need to reach and maintain a healthy weight.

Origins

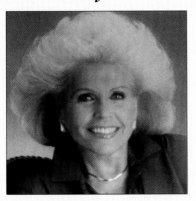

WEIGHT WATCHER PIONEER
Founder of Weight Watchers, Jean Nidetch could not have predicted its huge and lasting success. In North America alone hundreds of thousands attend meetings each week.

By age 38, Jean Nidetch weighed 97 kg (214 lb) but secretly despised her condition. She soothed her low self-esteem with cycles of overeating and crash dieting. In 1961 she began attending an Obesity Clinic and, following a low-cholesterol, calorie-controlled diet, attained a sustainable weight of 64 kg (141 lb). She linked her success with being able to talk over her problems with friends each week and recognizing how emotional problems can lead to unhealthy eating habits. In 1963 she founded Weight Watchers in New York to help others to achieve similar results.

A leader of a commercial weight-loss club is a person who has been trained to conduct weekly meetings on behalf of the organization. To qualify for training he or she must have completed a successful weight-loss program with the organization and then maintained a target weight. A group leader thus provides a positive role model who understands the whole experience of being overweight and changing one's lifestyle to lose weight. Training covers basic principles of psychology and health, as well as advanced skills of behavior modification and group interaction and communication. Such leaders are generally adept at guiding and motivating members to produce and maintain lifestyle changes of their own.

How do I join a club?

The parent organization of your chosen club can tell you where the nearest meeting center is. Meetings are usually held weekly, and you should have no trouble finding a time to suit you. Some groups will even come to an office if enough people sign up to attend sessions.

What happens at group meetings?

The leader will register your membership (although with some clubs you don't have to join until after the first meeting), introduce you to fellow group members, and weigh you. Your weight is confidential and remains so throughout the program. Sessions center around group discussions of the issues and problems surrounding weight loss and dieting. Group leaders use their training to coordinate and guide the discussions, as well as teaching behavioral techniques to help members reform their eating habits. Although members do tend to discuss with each other how they are doing, confidentiality about each person's actual weight and the number of pounds he or she has lost is observed at all times.

Every week your weight loss progress is checked, and group members discuss their own progress and problems, talk about their methods, and exchange tips. The leader provides support and advice on many aspects of nutrition and exercise. There may even be demonstrations of calorie-controlled recipes or slimming products, possibly with pressure to buy.

How do I figure out how much weight to lose?

Setting realistic goals and a sensible personal agenda for weight loss is an extremely important step, and your group leader will give you as much guidance as possible. The leader will have charts and tables that are used to work out your ideal healthy weight range, but you will set your own targets. This means that you can choose to lose as little as 3 kg (6 lb 8 oz) or as much as you believe necessary to reach your ideal weight. The club will support whatever you decide as long as your weight goal is within the healthy range for your height.

How do I actually lose weight in a dieting club?

Many clubs work on a point system. They provide comprehensive food lists and tables in which a score is allocated to various foodstuffs, based on their caloric value. You are allotted a points budget for each day, which is based on your age, sex, starting weight, and activity levels. The budget is set at a level that will guarantee your calorie expenditure exceeds your intake. Within this budget you are free to eat whatever you like, although healthy eating guidelines such as lowering levels of fat and cholesterol should also be considered. There may even be a list of very-low-calorie foods, of which you can eat unlimited amounts. You will have to keep a record of what you've eaten, so that your points tally can be calculated. In some cases, points can be saved for special occasions or earned through exercise. The basic theme of the weight control plan is to achieve a diet that is balanced and full of variety.

Do I have to exercise?

Different clubs have varying philosophies about exercise. Most will encourage you to become more active, but few actually include exercise routines as part of the weekly sessions. In most clubs, you can earn points by doing exercise.

Can anyone join?

Young persons under 16 will need permission from a doctor. People whose Body Mass Index shows that they are underweight will not be allowed to join, and anyone with a health condition should obtain a doctor's consent before starting a slimming program.

How long do most weight-loss programs last?

Obviously this will depend on how much weight you aim to lose and how well you manage to stick to the diet plan you are given. The maximum healthy weight loss per week is 0.5 to 1 kg (1 to 2 lb). If you are losing more than this you should have a medical check-up, and it may be necessary to come off the diet.

Do organizations provide support to people who have reached their target weight?

Yes. To help you maintain your weight loss you will probably be welcome to continue attending meetings, perhaps even free of charge, and encouraged to help motivate others. Alternatively, you may be given a program to take home that contains advice on how to maintain your new weight.

Are there any regulatory bodies for these dieting clubs?

There is no official regulatory body, but any weight loss claims made in advertisements or promotional literature are bound by certain regulations. Reputable organizations prepare their diets and food plans along the recommended guidelines on nutrition, diet, and weight control.

WHAT YOU CAN DO AT HOME

It is a good idea to supplement your membership in a weight-loss club with a home exercise program. As most clubs don't include exercise in their weight plans, following your own regimen will help you consolidate your achievements in the class, and can even earn you points for your calorie budget. Some people find exercise videos helpful, particularly if they have never attended formal exercise classes or are worried about exercising in the company of others. You can do aerobic exercises in the privacy of your own living room and take things at your own pace. To come to grips with the exercises on the screen, you can replay movements that you find difficult until you've mastered them. Making up your own exercises is not advisable. All the ones chosen for home workouts are usually easy to copy, and if you follow them carefully you should not injure yourself. A good video starts with a series of warm-up exercises before moving on to a comprehensive routine that works all the major muscle groups. For your own motivation, look for a video that is led by someone who personally inspires you or who is well-known and respected in the field of health and fitness.

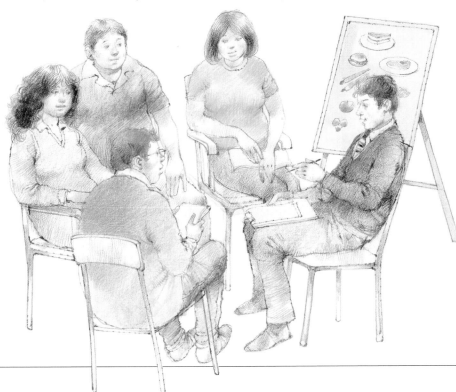

PRIVATE CLINICS

Private weight-loss clinics can be a lifesaving experience for anyone who is severely obese and has had no success with other programs. Most operate under the guidance of one or more physicians and dietitians who closely monitor the dieter's health. If they have any drawbacks it is that some of them accept in their care individuals who may be only mildly overweight or do not need to lose weight at all,

HEALTH CLUBS

Many dieters are helped by health clubs that emphasize physical activity. Most provide the necessary advice and support for people at all levels of fitness and offer a wide range of activities from which to choose. Included usually are weight training, gym workouts, aerobic classes, and swimming, all of which can have positive effects on the mind and body. There is considerable evidence that an increased level of physical activity is one of the best ways to prevent weight gain, especially after a period of successful weight loss, but it is difficult to lose weight through exercise alone without changing your diet. Unfortunately, many health clubs do not provide qualified dietary advice to members. Another drawback is that some of them can be quite expensive. Look for those that offer special rates at off-peak times.

HEALTH FARMS

There are now many health farms, or spas (see page 113), that offer the chance to relax in a pleasant environment equipped with everything necessary for relaxation and weight loss. Healthful, balanced meals, exercise programs, and special treatments such as massage are provided, and many people see this as a welcome break from the stresses of everyday living. However, health spas are usually a very expensive way to lose weight, and there is no guarantee that a short stay in this environment will help you change the bad habits of a lifetime.

BEHAVIOR THERAPY GROUPS

For many overweight individuals, psychological factors associated with obesity have to be overcome for weight loss to be successful and permanent, especially when food is used to cope with boredom, loneliness, insecurity, and frustrations. Old habits are difficult to change, but many weight-loss groups now use behavioral therapy to try to alter eating habits. Large weight-control organizations such as Weight Watchers also use elements of behavioral modification techniques in their programs. People who have tried behavior modification on their own and failed may benefit from group therapy, but it is worth checking the credentials of the professionals involved in any program. Some group leaders do not have adequate qualifications. If you're in doubt, your doctor or dietitian may be able to suggest a suitable behavior modification center.

The aim of behavior therapy is to help people identify negative factors that encourage bad eating habits and replace these with more healthful patterns. Dieters are encouraged to keep food and activity diaries, remove foods that may precipitate binge eating from the home and workplace, and pay more attention to the act of eating. Once the pitfalls have been identified, a plan can be adapted to suit an individual's needs. Dieters are taught to reward themselves for positive behavior, rather than weight loss.

Being with other people in a similar situation can also have a positive impact on behavior. New perspective is gained from learning about the ways in which others have motivated themselves or have overcome failure. Weight loss can occur if the dieter follows a calorie-restricted diet, but changing behavior can enhance motivation and help make this easier to achieve.

Some weight-loss groups also employ meditation techniques or hypnosis to try to change eating habits. These methods may help people relax and deal positively with everyday tensions that induce overeating, provided they are carried out by trained specialists. However, there is no concrete proof that these approaches induce significant weight loss. Adequate dietary advice is crucial to long-term success in any weight-loss program that employs behavior therapy.

It has been suggested that behavioral methods should be applied to an entire family, not just an overweight individual. Studies have verified that weight loss is more likely to be successful for a subject whose spouse or other family members participate actively in treatment. The treatment offered should still be based on sound nutritional principles, but the insights that the family gains can contribute greatly to the success of the person trying to lose weight.

STEP-BY-STEP FITNESS Joining a health club or an aerobics class may be an expense, but the professional guidance will help you avoid injury and get the most out of your time. It will also provide ongoing support and possibly increase your motivation.

CHAPTER 8

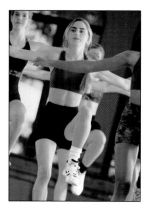

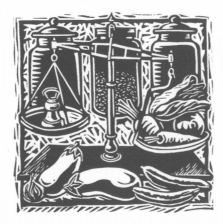

YOUR WEIGHT-CONTROL PLAN

The secret of a successful weight-control plan is to tailor your diet and exercise regimens to suit your own needs. This means looking at your lifestyle both at home and at work and setting realistic goals that take into account existing demands on your time and energy.

STARTING A WEIGHT-CONTROL PROGRAM

If it is to be successful, a weight-control program needs to be introduced with care, setting a realistic long-term goal and establishing ways to keep motivated.

Earlier chapters have discussed the extent to which people's ideas of ideal weight are shaped by outside forces: advertising and the media set goals that are impossible for most people to attain. If your own goal is to end up with the same statistics as a catwalk model, you are probably destined to be disappointed. It is enlightening to realize that this body shape is natural for only 5 percent of the population.

Your ideal weight should be based on a combination of your age, body mass index, or BMI, and body shape. Once you establish which shape you are, you can form a more reasonable ideal weight goal.

FINDING YOUR IDEAL WEIGHT

If you are an endomorph or a mesomorph (see box, below) you will need to accept that your natural body shape is more rounded, and that basing a weight-control plan on the tall, thin body image of a fashion model—the typical ectomorph—will not be very attainable. Fixing your sights on this body image is likely to lead to a constant weight battle that is ultimately doomed to failure. It may be more helpful to focus on a role model—such as an actor, TV personality, or show-business celebrity—who is closer to your own height and build and who has a figure that you admire.

KNOWING YOUR BODY SHAPE

Most people fit more or less into one of three body-type categories: endomorph, mesomorph, or ectomorph. Establishing which is your shape can help you develop an exercise plan that targets the areas where you are most likely to put on weight. While you can't change the way your body type distributes fat, you can firm up muscles in the problem areas to give you a more defined shape.

Endomorphs should target the abdominal muscles to tone the stomach, while mesomorphs (the category most women fall into) should concentrate on the thighs and buttocks. The tall, slim ectomorphs should give equal attention to all the major muscle groups.

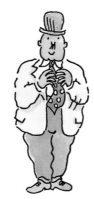

ENDOMORPHS (APPLE-SHAPED PEOPLE)
They tend to put on weight around their stomachs and waists. Their legs are often shorter than their torsos and they are shorter than average in stature.

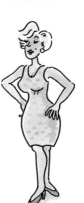

MESOMORPHS (PEAR-SHAPED PEOPLE)
Mesomorphs have hips wider than their shoulders and legs that are about the same length as their torsos. Weight is usually gained around the thighs, then hips and buttocks.

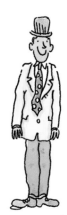

ECTOMORPHS (BEAN-POLE SHAPED PEOPLE)
They are taller, with long legs in proportion to their torsos. Any excess weight is usually evenly distributed over the body. Most fashion models are ectomorphs.

Achieving your goals

Before embarking on your weight plan you need to accept the fact that results are not going to be instantaneous. Successful, long-term weight loss comes from gradual change that can be maintained over a long period of time, not crash diets that bring about only temporary weight loss. Your goal will best be achieved by reorienting yourself to new ways of eating and exercising that you can practice for the rest of your life. First, however, you have to prepare yourself for the changes that this new approach will bring to your present situation.

Your lifestyle and needs

Remember that your ideal weight should take into account the demands that your lifestyle places on you. If you lead a particularly active life—for example, if you are a teacher chasing after young children all day—you need more energy than a sedentary office worker to function effectively. However, even a sedentary person requires energy to maintain his activities (see page 130 for calculating caloric needs). A weight-control plan should never mean starving yourself, but rather it should involve changing the types of food you eat.

Until now a large proportion of your energy may have been supplied by high-fat foods at mealtimes. In addition, you may have snacked on cookies, pastries, or chocolate bars that are high in fat and sugar to give yourself a short-term energy boost. Now you should aim to reduce your fat and sugar intake gradually and to increase the complex carbohydrates in your diet from foods such as bread, rice, and pasta. They will provide energy in a less concentrated form than fat, but the energy will be more slowly released in the body than that from simple sugar—the kind prevalent in sweets. This means the energy will be readily accessible and sustain you for longer periods.

WHICH DIET IF ANY?

Deciding to begin a weight-control program doesn't necessarily mean starting a diet. The word itself often conjures up images of lettuce leaves, carrots, and starvation. In fact some studies suggest that strict dieting can encourage people to become obsessive about food, which may, in turn, lead to overeating. One study conducted in the United States in the 1950s examined the effects of dieting on 36 men who were put on a calorie-controlled plan that reduced their food intake by approximately half over a 12-week period. While all of the men lost weight, it was observed that some members of the group became fixated on food to the point that they began to steal or hoard it. They also became depressed and apathetic. A follow-up study after the period of dieting revealed a pattern of bingeing and loss of control over their eating habits.

Highly restrictive dieting can be counter-productive and is not the best route to effective weight management. Successful weight control involves becoming better informed about food and nutrition, and particularly about fat, so that eating habits change permanently. When most people examine their current eating patterns they find that they could fairly easily cut down on the amount of fat and sugar they eat to reduce the total number of calories they consume each day. Sometimes this is all that is needed. If they make permanent changes in their eating habits and establish and stick to a regular routine of exercise, they lose weight without undertaking a more formalized diet or reducing their volume of food.

Some people, however, find that they need the discipline of a diet plan to keep them focused and motivated. Others require an initial drastic change in eating habits to introduce long-term change. If this is the case for you, make sure that you assess the

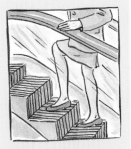

QUICK FITNESS TIP
Each time you use an escalator, walk up instead of letting the escalator do the leg work for you. Better still, use the stairs.

BURNING OFF CALORIES: *Rowing*

Rowing, either using a machine in the gym or a boat on water, is an excellent aerobic exercise. It puts all your body's major muscle groups to work and develops endurance.

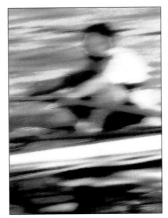

MUSCLE GROUPS BENEFITING
Rowing exercises muscles in your legs, chest, arms, abdomen, shoulders, back, and buttocks.

EQUIPMENT
A sturdy rowing machine or a small rowboat.

CALORIES BURNED
During rowing, you expend an average of 11 calories per minute: that's 660 calories per hour.

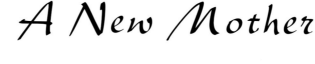

A New Mother

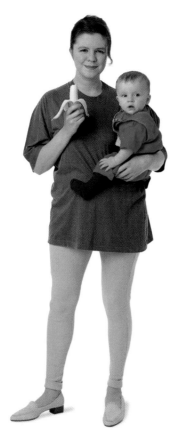

A young baby can quickly sabotage a new mother's well-laid plans for getting back to prepregnancy weight and shape. There are constant demands on time and energy, together with the exhausting effects of interrupted sleep. These make it hard to find the resources to exercise or the will to prepare healthy meals. Convenience foods and snacks may be all you have time for or feel up to, with the result that you fail to shed the weight you put on during pregnancy and cannot regain your previous shape. Remember that your body has specific nutritional needs during breastfeeding and you should not diet during this time, but you can still begin a healthier eating plan.

FOOD

PROBLEM 1
No time to cook proper meals
When you are rushed off your feet looking after a young baby, cooking proper meals may seem like a luxury. Instead you rely on convenience meals and processed foods.

SOLUTION
Try to get more support. Friends, family members and neighbors are often delighted to help, so don't feel you have to do everything yourself. Use the extra time to prepare some healthy meals. Follow the basic rules of cutting down on fat and increasing fruit and vegetable intake. If your baby is eating solids you could purée some of your meal for him to share. Remember, variety is a good way to make sure that both you and your child get all the nutrients you need.

PROBLEM 2
Sugary or high-fat snacks
Fatigue can leave you feeling lethargic, run-down, and in need of an immediate energy boost from sweets and high-fat snacks.

SOLUTION
Turn snacking to your advantage. More and smaller meals each day may be better than a few large ones. Eat high fiber, low-fat, low-sugar snacks; these will fill you up without adding too many calories. For an energy boost, eat a banana, which is high in potassium, a mineral essential for muscle and nerve function; or try a handful of raisins, which are high in iron but low in fat.

LIFESTYLE

PROBLEM 1
No time or energy to exercise
If you haven't kept up with your postnatal exercises, your muscles won't have toned and you will feel too tired to move on to aerobic exercise. Although a baby is a constant demand on your time, finding ways of exercising together can be stimulating for you both.

SOLUTION
Increasing activity levels will help you obtain a net calorie loss, while toning exercises will tighten your muscles, thus improving your figure. Though you may feel too tired to do any exercise it is worth persevering, because in the long run your energy levels will increase. Involve your baby in your postnatal exercises; start by walking with the child in a carriage or sling. Swimming is another aerobic exercise that you can both enjoy by joining a mother and baby class. Many pools also have childcare facilities, so that you can swim a few laps on your own.

PROBLEM 2
Lack of sleep
The new baby disrupts your sleep, depleting your energy and leaving you tense and exhausted.

SOLUTION
Practice some relaxation techniques whenever you have a few free moments. Meditation, visualization, or yoga can help your body recover from the fatigue of disrupted sleep and give you more energy.

CUTTING CALORIES

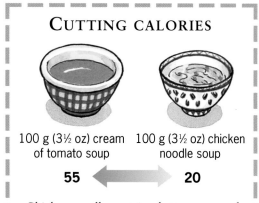

100 g (3½ oz) cream of tomato soup

55 ⬅➡ **20**

100 g (3½ oz) chicken noodle soup

Chicken noodle soup is a better source of fiber and protein and is also more filling.

benefits before you start a diet to ensure that you have made the right choice (see Chapter 7). Remember that a diet must follow sound nutritional guidelines by including all the major food groups and the vital vitamins and minerals.

Carefully assess any published health risks and other research for evidence about the diet's efficacy before you begin. Discuss your findings with your doctor so that together you can consider how the diet might affect you. It may be that the plan can be adapted slightly so that it suits your particular needs. Remember, for successful long-term weight management, a diet should encourage healthier eating habits that can be continued after your target weight has been reached. Examine the technical demands of the diet, such as weighing food and counting calories, and ask yourself if you will be able to stick to it in the long term. Another important aspect to consider is whether the diet is within your budget and if you can successfully adapt your lifestyle to follow it.

Pathway to health

Natural therapies are of particular help if your eating habits are influenced by your emotions. Stress can play a major role in inducing bad habits like comfort eating and snacking on the run, which can be responsible for weight gain. Introducing relaxation techniques such as meditation or reflexology into your daily life (see Chapter 6) may help you break a cycle of high-fat snacking or bingeing.

For example, can it be worked in with your partner's eating habits or your children's dietary needs?

Whatever dietary changes you make or whatever diet you follow, you should also consider introducing more exercise into your life. Most experts agree that exercise combined with diet provides the best results for long-term weight loss and maintenance of reduced weight (see Chapter 5).

The psychology of diets

Studies have shown that many dieters fail when they develop an obsessive attitude about following the diet. If you feel that you have blown the diet completely by eating one chocolate bar, you are susceptible to binge eating. Try to avoid becoming obsessive and forgive yourself for the occasional slip up. It is difficult to maintain rigid eating controls at all times.

If you understand the principles of healthy eating and exercise, and realize that having a three-course restaurant meal one night may mean smaller servings of food the next day or a longer period of exercise, you will be able to master the eating challenges everyone faces from time to time. If your weight goal is set to be achieved within a realistic period of time, one or two incidents of breaking the rules will have little fundamental effect. As long as you make the effort to return to your plan and don't use occasional faltering as an excuse to give up, your goal will still be attainable.

MOTIVATION

Try to keep a positive outlook while you establish your weight-control plan. As well as keeping focused on your long-term goal, set yourself interim goals that are well within your abilities to achieve. For instance, set a small target weight loss of 2.5 kg (5½ lb) at the end of the first three weeks of your diet and exercise program.

Set dietary goals too. Aim to eat an extra piece of fruit each day or to stop taking sugar in tea and coffee. Small goals are important, because they can keep you motivated even when weight loss seems slow. Any step in the right direction will help toward achieving long-term goals.

Be sure to praise yourself for all of your successes and to record them in a diary or notebook (see right) that you can refer to whenever you need a psychological boost.

RECORDING YOUR PROGRESS

Keeping a diary during your weight-management plan can help you remain positive and determined. You may go through a week in which you do not lose any weight at all, but can be spurred on by reminding yourself of your successes so far. The most obvious entry is your weekly weight reading, but there are several other things you could record:

▶ *The results of the step test (see page 84).*

▶ *Your waist-hip ratio (see page 24).*

▶ *Positive feedback such as flattering comments regarding your appearance.*

▶ *Feelings of increased well-being.*

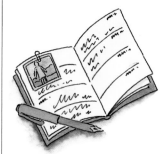

PHOTOGRAPHIC EVIDENCE
Include a photograph in your diary so that you can see how far you have come since you began your weight-control program. See page 129 for how to set up a suitable snapshot.

Rather than weighing yourself obsessively, set exercise targets that you have to meet, and take pride in watching your fitness levels develop. As your fitness increases you will have the satisfaction of knowing that your muscles are being toned, your general health and vitality getting better, and your metabolic rate increasing. All of these factors will improve your general appearance and you will feel an increased sense of well-being. These changes should prove that you are making progress.

Find ways to make food control fun

Try different healthy snacks to discover the ones you really enjoy, and make sure you turn to them when you feel the emotional need for comfort eating, rather than to high-fat or high-sugar snacks and sweets. This will help you keep to your weight-control program, and you will be less likely to lapse during times of emotional crisis.

You should also adjust the way you view the dietary changes you have adopted, so that they add fun and interest to your life, instead of making dieting seem like a chore. All good diet plans recommend including more fruit and vegetables in your meals, so try new produce, giving yourself the occasional exotic treat. For example experiment with a new vegetable to liven up your main courses. Plantains might make a substitute for potatoes. They vary in flavor as they ripen, from potato to sweet potato, and can be cooked in the same way as regular potatoes. Celeriac, or celery root, can be boiled, fried, stewed, or used in salads.

There is also a whole range of unusual fruits that you could try for dessert or as a healthy snack. A custard apple, or cherimoya, which looks like an oversized green pinecone, has creamy, custard-flavored flesh and is a good source of vitamin C. Persimmon, a popular autumn fruit that is increasingly available, has a complex, sweet flavor. Others to consider include guava (available in fall and early winter), litchee nut (found in Asian markets in summer), and carambola, or star fruit. A selection of these fruits could be used to make an exotic fruit salad.

INCREASING YOUR MOTIVATION

A weight-loss plan that is built around a low-fat diet and regular exercise to improve your level of fitness will lead to many health benefits as well as helping with weight loss. You will feel more energetic and healthy as you progress with your regimen. You will also be lowering your risk of many chronic diseases, including coronary heart disease and cancer. These are all important reasons for losing weight, but you may need other spurs to boost your determination, willpower, and self-motivation.

▶ *Find a photograph of yourself when you were slimmer. Keep it prominently displayed as a reminder of what you can achieve.*

▶ *Add a partner to your plan, your mate or a friend who shares your long-term goal. Establish an exercise regimen together and share tips on recipes and low-fat shopping.*

▶ *Enlist your family's support: dieting will be much easier if they share in your new healthy, low-fat approach, or at the very least don't undermine your efforts.*

▶ *Each time you chart considerable progress in weight loss or fitness, give yourself a reward: buy a new item of clothing or some flowers, or plan an outing to a favorite place.*

▶ *Keep exercise clothing and equipment near at hand, so that you don't miss any sessions because you forgot or couldn't get organized. Keeping your running shoes beside the bed, for example, can serve as a useful prod.*

▶ *Stop thinking negatively and instead focus your mind on the improvements that you have made so far. Start each day with a positive affirmation or two such as "Today I will eat well, feel great, and look better than ever." This is called autosuggestion (see page 97) and can go a long way toward improving your self-esteem and motivation.*

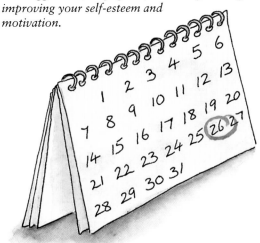

SETTING A TARGET DATE TO AIM FOR
Set down the date of an event or engagement to provide you with a weight-loss goal to work toward: something that is not unrealistically soon, but is four or five months away and is important to you. It could be perhaps a special holiday that you want to be fit and healthy for or a friend's wedding.

A Retired Person

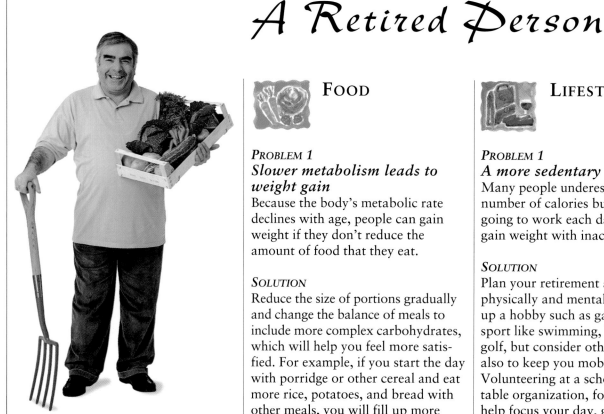

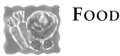 ## FOOD

PROBLEM 1
Slower metabolism leads to weight gain
Because the body's metabolic rate declines with age, people can gain weight if they don't reduce the amount of food that they eat.

SOLUTION
Reduce the size of portions gradually and change the balance of meals to include more complex carbohydrates, which will help you feel more satisfied. For example, if you start the day with porridge or other cereal and eat more rice, potatoes, and bread with other meals, you will fill up more quickly and consume less.

PROBLEM 2
Less money to spend on food
For many people retirement can mean less to spend on food, leading to purchases of more high-fat processed foods. Reduced mobility can also affect the types of foods bought.

SOLUTION
Eating low-fat and nutritious food doesn't have to be expensive. Canned fish, for instance, is generally affordable and provides generous amounts of protein. Eating more fruits and vegetables and less meat will save you money and provide important vitamins and minerals. Because many fruits and vegetables lose some of their nutrients when processed, it is better to buy them fresh or quick frozen or grow your own. Many stores will deliver, if transportation and mobility are a problem.

 ## LIFESTYLE

PROBLEM 1
A more sedentary lifestyle
Many people underestimate the number of calories burned simply by going to work each day and find they gain weight with inactivity.

SOLUTION
Plan your retirement around staying physically and mentally active. Take up a hobby such as gardening or a sport like swimming, bowling, or golf, but consider other activities also to keep you mobile and active. Volunteering at a school or charitable organization, for example, can help focus your day, get you out of the house, and prevent the boredom that can lead to snacking. Use your extra free time to walk more often: to the local stores or to visit friends.

PROBLEM 2
Exercise is painful
The onset of arthritis and other age-related illnesses can discourage people from exercise.

SOLUTION
Although exercise may be painful at first, it is particularly beneficial for arthritis sufferers. Doing warm-up stretches before exercising can reduce pain. Ask your doctor for advice on exercise options. A non-weight-bearing activity such as swimming can ease the strain on joints, while a weight-bearing one like walking can help strengthen bones. Massage can also help loosen joints before exercise and ease any pain afterward.

Weight can be a problem for many retired people, because they have to overcome a number of potential threats to their waistlines. Not only does metabolism slow down with age, making the body slower at burning energy, but also retirement can lead to less activity, and, at the same time, arthritis and other age-related illnesses can make exercise difficult. A reduced income may mean you have to compromise on food. Planting a vegetable garden can provide both fresh vegetables and regular exercise. Many older people find themselves eating alone and don't make as much effort to cook fresh food. With careful planning, however, retirement does not have to lead to weight gain.

123

YOUR EATING HABITS

Changing eating patterns takes determination and motivation. First you need to assess honestly what you currently eat and then find ways to improve your habits at work and at home.

In order to make a permanent change in your eating habits, you need to assess what and when you normally eat. Armed with this information, you can decide whether these food habits are conducive to reaching and maintaining your ideal weight.

WHAT YOU REALLY EAT

As discussed in Chapter 4, effective weight management is largely about controlling the amount of fat in a diet. However, many people remain ignorant about how much fat they actually eat. It is easy to convince yourself that your current diet is reasonably healthy, unless you take the time to list everything you eat and examine the fat content. Keep a food diary for a week (see page 47), noting exactly what you ate and when you ate it. Use the food charts on pages 66–67, plus other information available in nutrition books and on food package labels, to determine the number of fat grams and calories in the food you have eaten. Then apply the fat formula on page 73 to work out what percentage of your diet is fat. The aim, of course, is to keep it at 30 percent or less of total daily intake. As much as possible familiarize yourself with products that are truly low in fat. Before long, buying healthy food will have become a habit.

RECOGNIZING YOUR DANGER TIMES

Snacking excessively between meals is the downfall of many people, even when they are eating carefully planned meals. In order to break the habit, it helps to understand the reasons behind it. Common causes include depression and boredom. Identifying the periods when you are most likely to reach for a high-fat snack will arm you in the battle to take control of such impulses. If, for instance, you see a pattern of snacking during especially stressful periods at work, force yourself to take a break rather than reaching for something to eat. Take the time to perform a few easy stretches or make a cup of tea. Even a brisk walk up and down stairs, around the office, or around the block can break your stress/food cycle.

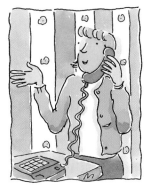

CHEER YOURSELF UP
There is often a link between snacking and being lonely, bored, or depressed. Rather than reaching for comfort food, find an activity, such as phoning or writing to a friend, that will lift your mood.

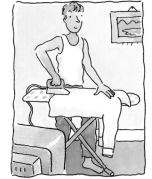

KEEP BUSY
If your danger period is at night while watching television, try to do something more active during this time. When there is a program you want to see, do something useful such as ironing while you watch TV, to keep yourself busy and prevent snacking.

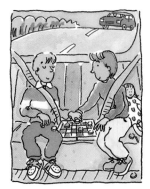

ALLEVIATE BOREDOM
If your children get bored during long journeys, don't placate them with sweets. Provide some travel games instead, or play games that involve spotting things along the road. Also, bring some fruit, so that you are prepared if they get hungry.

A Young Family

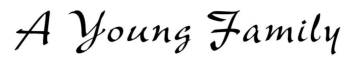

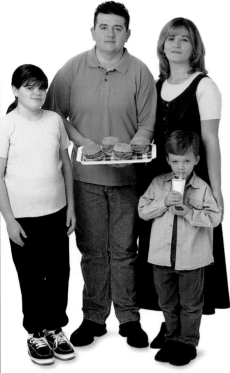

I f you have a family you may find it difficult to initiate new eating habits for yourself without changing their habits at the same time. The least successful diets are those that require people to eat in isolation from their families, cooking one meal for themselves and another for the other members. Because low-fat foods are not only better for controlling weight but also contribute to good health, changing dietary habits is important for the entire family. Aim to change your family's preferences for high-sugar and high-fat foods and enlist their support for your long-term goals.

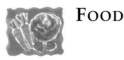 FOOD

PROBLEM 1
Nutrition needs for children
Your own low-fat diet may create unforeseen nutritional problems for your children.

SOLUTION
Because children are still growing, they should not have their calorie intakes restricted, but it is important to introduce them to healthy eating habits at the same time as you are improving your own. Make sure that they are getting the necessary calcium and other nutrients for growth by adapting your own meals for them. Keep a supply of whole milk for the children and low-fat or skim milk for yourself. Add cheese for them to low-fat salads that you prepare for yourself. If you are serving baked potatoes, make fillings more calorie-rich for the children with creamy sauces, while you fill your own with water-packed tuna or yogurt.

PROBLEM 2
Finicky eating
Your children and perhaps your partner resist or oppose changes to their favorite meals.

SOLUTION
Adjusting your family's favorite recipes by reducing fat whenever possible is a way of subtly changing habits. Also, make hamburgers healthier by using extra-lean meat and serving them on whole-wheat buns. Gradually cut down the amount of sugar in desserts that you prepare and in other items you buy.

LIFESTYLE

PROBLEM 1
Lazy family habits
The family as a whole may prefer watching television to sports and other physical activities.

SOLUTION
Gradually wean everyone away from the television. Begin by playing board games, then move on to more active pursuits that are also fun such as swimming or roller-blading.

PROBLEM 2
Your partner doesn't support your plan
If your partner is overweight, he or she may have a vested interest in keeping you plump. A partner may even sabotage your best efforts by bringing home treats of chocolate or cake or take-out food, to relieve you of the burden of cooking.

SOLUTION
Discuss your goals with your partner. Make sure he or she understands the importance of what you are trying to do and some of the principles of healthy, low-fat eating and exercise that you are attempting to introduce. Get your partner involved in menu planning and exercise ideas. Perhaps he or she has a favorite sport you could share.

If your partner brings home treats, try to maintain your self control. Explain that these make your task harder and, though the occasional treat is fine, if this happens on a regular basis it will undermine your careful eating plan.

Low-fat cooking

You can cut fat in many small ways each day, and, when you add them up, the total can be significant. For example, use low-fat spreads instead of regular butter or margarine whenever possible. Boil, poach, or scramble eggs rather than frying them. Choose tuna canned in water rather than oil. Substitute low-fat or nonfat sour cream or yogurt for butter on baked potatoes and for cream to accompany fruit. Choose sorbet or low-fat frozen yogurt for dessert rather than ice cream. If you can't eliminate cake completely from your diet, cut back on those that have icing or whipped cream and look for ones that gain some of their moisture from fruit rather than butter. Adjust the way you cook and prepare foods as well. For example, grate cheese for sandwiches rather than cutting slices; you will use less. Instead of frying food, grill, broil, steam, or poach it. When you do fry, use a nonstick pan and minimal oil and drain the food on absorbent paper to remove any excess fat.

MEAL PLANNING

Most successful dieters report that a major part of their accomplishment was due to eating regular meals and carefully considering their content to maximize necessary nutrients and taste, while minimizing unnecessary fat. If your existing diet is high in fat, you may have to check the fat and calorie contents of every food until low-fat eating becomes second nature to you. As you start to exert greater control over what you eat, build your meals around filling, low-fat complex carbohydrates that will diminish

Pathway to health
As you become involved in creating a healthier diet you may enjoy trying new recipes and exploring the cuisines of different cultures. You could contact a local high school or college for a schedule of adult courses in cooking. Vegetarian, Italian, Chinese, and Japanese cuisines can all be low in fat. You may find that attending classes also spurs your motivation and lifts your mood, as well as providing a new skill with which to entertain your friends.

your hunger pangs, as well as giving you the right levels of energy. Pasta dishes, crusty whole-grain bread, baked potatoes with their skins, and brown rice all create a satisfied feeling and keep your body well fueled.

INTRODUCING CHANGES

For many people the stumbling block to changing eating habits is taste. If you have for years been eating predominantly fatty or sugary foods, changing your habits is going to mean changing your food preferences. The best way to do this is gradually, giving your body time to adjust to reductions rather than immediately cutting out all your preferred foods. If a favorite meal is high in fat, first try to reduce the frequency with which you eat that meal. If you regularly buy a take-out treat, think about cooking the same meal at home. For example, hamburgers, french fries, and pizzas, can all be made at home with healthier, lower-calorie ingredients and cooking methods. Next, try to cut down on the amount you eat; portion sizes of take-out food are often much larger than you would prepare in your own kitchen.

If you have a sweet tooth, cutting back on sugar may be the most difficult change to make. Start by serving fresh fruit with your regular ice-cream. Then serve fruit with flavored yogurt, gradually changing to low-fat, plain yogurt as you develop a taste for less sugar. Instead of denying yourself sweets totally, have an occasional small portion of something really special like a rich cake or chocolate truffle. Eliminate soft drinks, even the types that contain an artificial sweetener. Some researchers believe that sugar substitutes actually heighten a craving for sweets.

HEALTHY "FRIED" FOODSS

It is possible to prepare healthful versions of fried foods by broiling and baking. These homemade chips were baked, in a single layer, on a nonstick baking sheet at 175°C/350° F for about 50 minutes. The fish was lightly coated with batter and broiled for about 4 minutes on each side.

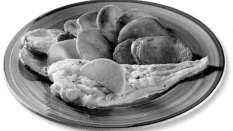

A LOW-FAT MEAL
Broiled and baked foods like this fish and chips can be enhanced by adding pepper, paprika, Parmesan, or lemon juice for extra tang.

An Office Worker

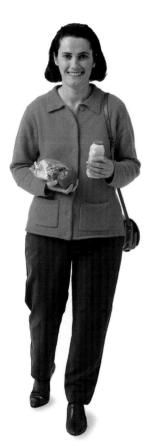

People who work most of their lives in an office perhaps don't realize how much their work environment can influence eating and exercise patterns. In general, office workers are seated for much of the day and have few opportunities for more activity. At the same time, they may find it hard to resist high-fat temptations from a vending machine or nearby delicatessen. Their will to eat healthfully can also be sorely tested by the snacking habits of co-workers and by expense-account lunches at restaurants or social occasions after work.

FOOD

PROBLEM 1
High-fat lunches
You may face temptations of high-calorie foods in a company cafeteria or from nearby sandwich shops and restaurants.

SOLUTION
Take time to study menus and work out the options that are lowest in fat. Look at sandwich and salad options rather than quiche or pies that will be high in fat because of their pastry content. Try to prepare your own lunch at least two or three times a week (see page 128). You can better control the nutritional content and will probably also save money. Choose high-fiber bread and high-protein, low-fat fillings such as grilled fish or skinless chicken. Use mustard or ketchup as a spread instead of mayonnaise or butter.

PROBLEM 2
Snacking during the day
It's easy to give yourself treats or energy boosts during the day that quickly add calories.

SOLUTION
Try beverages such as herbal tea or mineral water as an alternative to food. If you must have a snack, make it fruit, low-fat crackers, or rice cakes. The natural sweetness of fruit will satisfy your craving for sweet foods, and the saving in calories and fat will be significant. Replacing a morning slice of coffee cake with two fresh plums will save over 150 calories and 5 g of fat.

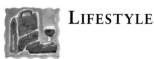

LIFESTYLE

PROBLEM 1
Lack of activity
If your job is largely desk-based, your metabolism may slow down during these long periods of inactivity, and you may find few opportunities for exercise.

SOLUTION
Use whatever free time you do have during the day for active pursuits. Set aside part of your lunchtime for some form of exercise. Organizing work colleagues to join you one day a week at a nearby gym might help motivate you to maintain your own exercise. On other days of the week, try to do at least a 20-minute brisk walk. You could also set up some office teams for sports such as football or softball after work.

PROBLEM 2
Boredom
If you work at your desk for most of the day and have a predictable work routine, you may become bored and use food as a diversion.

SOLUTION
Take regular breaks from sitting at your desk to stretch your muscles (see page 30) and refocus your eyes away from the computer screen or paperwork. These measures not only relieve tedium but also help prevent problems such as repetitive stress syndrome. Try discussing with your manager ways to vary your duties or increase your responsibilities. This will relieve boredom and distract you from a craving for snacks.

Packed Lunches

Much of the success of weight management rests on consistently controlling what you eat. Taking your own lunch to work allows you to limit your calorie intake, whereas visiting local eateries can tempt you into eating high-fat foods.

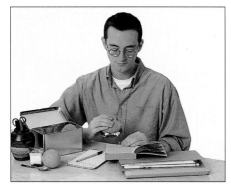

TAKING TIME OUT
Take a break from work at lunchtime to enjoy the food you have prepared.

Sandwiches are the obvious choice for a light, nutritious lunch at work. When making your own, limit your fat intake by avoiding butter and margarine altogether, or substitute a low-fat spread and spread it thinly or on one slice of bread only.

Breads can be an important source of fiber, protein, and iron, but they vary in fat and calorie content. Whole-grain bread, packed with fiber and vitamins, is the healthiest choice, while breads like foccacia that have a high oil content should be avoided.

THE CALORIE AND FAT CONTENT OF BREAD PER 100 g

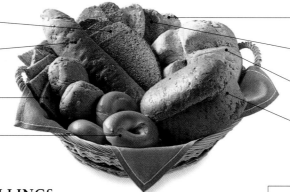

Pumpernickel = 221 calories, 0.9 g fat

Baguette = 258 calories, 1.5 g fat

Rye = 219 calories, 1.7 g fat

White bagel = 275 calories, 1.5 g fat

White pita = 265 calories, 1.2 g fat

Whole-wheat pita = 223 calories, 1.7 g fat

Cracked-wheat sourdough = 258 calories, 2.5 g fat

Seven-grain loaf = 235 calories, 2.7 g fat

LOW-FAT SANDWICH FILLINGS

When selecting sandwich fillers, consider the consistency of the bread to avoid a soggy and unappetizing lunch. Pack wet vegetables such as tomatoes and cucumbers separately and add them at the last minute, so they will not soak the bread. Try the following combinations:

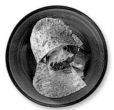

Grated cheese, grated carrot, and spinach leaves on pita bread = about 373 calories

Lean honey-cured ham, lettuce, and sun-dried tomato paste on a baguette = about 171 calories

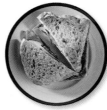

Smoked turkey, arugula leaves, and mango chutney on seven-grain bread = about 170 calories

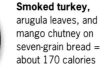

Sardines, green beans, and raddichio on cracked-wheat sourdough bread = about 277 calories

SALAD LUNCHES

Salad lunches make an ideal alternative to sandwiches. Buy low-fat cheese, cherry tomatoes, and shredded salad greens and add leftovers. For example, if you are cooking broccoli or beans for the evening meal, cook some extra to put in your salad the next day. Accompany the salad with a whole-grain bun.

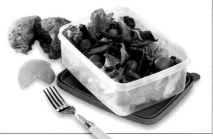

SELF-ASSESSMENT

Once your weight-control plan is successfully underway, monitoring your progress will permit you to see how well the program is working.

You should keep track of the rate at which you are losing weight, aiming for a gradual reduction: a weight loss of 0.5 to 1 kg (1 to 2 lb) a week is a sensible goal. If you lose in excess of 2 kg (4.5 lb) a week, you are losing weight too fast and should moderate your program or risk compromising your health. It is also important that you recognize when you should stop trying to lose weight and concentrate on weight maintenance instead.

GAUGING YOUR SUCCESS
For most people the scales are the ultimate arbiter of whether their weight-control plan has been successful or not. But scales can be a source of tyranny. While it is useful to check progress in this way, be reasonable in your expectations. Don't weigh yourself more than once or twice a week and bear in mind that early rapid weight loss, while encouraging, is likely to be largely fluid loss. Sustained weight loss, when stored supplies of fat begin to be used by the body, will take longer to occur.

Weight alone is not the only guide to progress in your new healthy lifestyle. If you have introduced an exercise program you should measure your increased levels of fitness as well. An improved resting heart rate and a better recovery rate from exercise (see page 79) are measurable and will show you when you have made progress in raising your metabolic rate and therefore are beginning to burn fat more quickly.

Even when the scales show that your weight is not falling, you may in fact have shed fat but have added muscle bulk. You can test whether or not your shape has changed by trying on tight-fitting skirts or trousers and seeing if they have loosened a little or hang any better.

On the other hand, be wary of gauging success in the mirror. You are not the most objective assessor of your own appearance. Evidence suggests that people distort the image they actually see in the mirror. Even someone in the healthy weight range for their age and height can perceive their mirror image to be overweight.

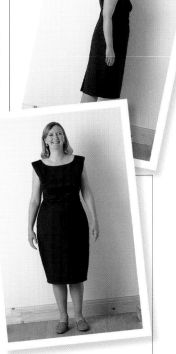

TELL-TALE ANGLES
Your shape looks different from the front and in profile; take one photo facing the camera and one sideways.

SETTING UP A SENSIBLE "BEFORE" SNAPSHOT

Weighing yourself is not the only way to judge the success of your weight-control regimen. For most people, looking slim and fitting easily into their clothes is the main motivation for dieting. A picture of yourself at the beginning of your plan will help boost your morale in the months ahead, when you see how much you have achieved. Here are some tips on setting up a realistic "before" photo:

▶ *If your camera has a self-timing mechanism, you can take the pictures yourself: set up the camera on a tripod or table top. Check the position by marking your height on the wall,*

or using an object the same height as yourself for a stand-in. Alternatively, ask a friend to take the picture for you.

▶ *Find an uncluttered background against which to take the photo so that there are no distractions from your figure. A blank wall is ideal; stand about a foot away from it.*

▶ *Wear close-fitting, plain-colored clothes. Patterns such as stripes and polkadots can cause optical illusions, making you appear bigger than you really are.*

▶ *Use a flash if possible. Otherwise, stand close to a window, so there is plenty of light, or take the picture outdoors.*

DANGER SIGNS OF EATING DISORDERS

Obsessive dieting can lead to eating disorders such as anorexia and bulimia. If you experience any of the danger signals listed below, consult your doctor immediately.

▶ *Missing three consecutive menstrual periods.*

▶ *Self-induced vomiting.*

▶ *Binge eating, especially of junk food, accompanied by mood swings.*

▶ *Food hoarding.*

▶ *Eating in secret.*

▶ *Depression and loss of sleep.*

▶ *Significant weight fluctuations—4.5 kg (10 lb) or more over a month.*

▶ *Dramatic weight loss over a short period of time.*

Unfortunately, this can be taken to extremes. Research conducted with anorexia nervosa sufferers has shown that they consistently see themselves as fatter than they actually are, to the point where young girls who are emaciated still see themselves in a mirror as being overweight. Rather than simply relying on the subjectivity of a mirror, gauge your success through things that are objectively measurable: weigh yourself, test your fitness level, and take your measurements.

As an alternative to the mirror, have a snapshot taken of yourself (see page 129) at the beginning of your weight-control program. After three months take a photograph wearing the same clothing and using the same lighting. The photographs can provide a more objective measurement of change. A photograph may also show you what part of your body you have a tendency to lose weight from first. These may be areas you have not been targeting. For example, a mesomorph woman (see page 118) may lose weight from her face and breasts rather than thighs and buttocks. Don't be disheartened if this is what your snapshot shows you. Be encouraged that you are losing weight and consider how to revise your exercise program to firm up problem areas.

Warning signs

If you are following a sensible, healthy eating plan and exercising, your diet will never become dangerous. It is when dieting becomes an obsession that you should step back and assess your behavior more objectively. If you feel fatigued and lethargic, this can be a sign that you are not eating enough to meet your caloric needs. Make sure that you have an adequate intake of complex carbohydrates to function properly.

Maintaining an ideal weight

Few people can or should maintain a diet severely controlled in calories. Successful dieters are those who sustain the broad principles of their weight-control plan. Remember, you can't return to old eating habits. Once you have lost weight your body needs less fuel to function efficiently. A rough rule of thumb is that for every pound of weight lost, you should eat 10 fewer calories. You can use the following formula as a guideline to determine roughly what your ideal weight is and then apply the guidelines on page 49 to figure how many calories you need.

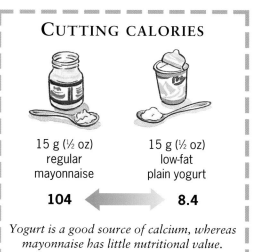

CUTTING CALORIES

15 g (½ oz)
regular
mayonnaise

15 g (½ oz)
low-fat
plain yogurt

104 ⟷ **8.4**

Yogurt is a good source of calcium, whereas mayonnaise has little nutritional value.

Females: Allow 100 pounds for the first 5 feet of height and 5 pounds per inch over 5 feet. For instance, if you are 5 feet, 5 inches tall (100 + 5 x 5 = 125 pounds). Add 5 to 10 pounds more if you are very muscular. **Males:** Allow 106 pounds for the first 5 feet of height and 6 pounds per inch over 5 feet. Thus, if you are 5 feet, 10 inches tall (106 + 10 x 6 = 166 pounds). Add 10 to 15 pounds more if you are very muscular.

FEELING CONTENT

As your eating habits improve and you start to exercise regularly you should soon feel and see the benefits to your body. The increased intake of vitamins C and A from fresh vegetables and fruit will improve your skin and exercise should improve your sleeping patterns, which will in turn help the restorative functions of the body. With a better flow of oxygen from exercise you will experience increased vitality and energy. Regular exercise will also firm and tone your muscles. All these factors should make you look and feel better than you did before you started. Even if you haven't met your target weight, you will have made substantial improvements to your health and well-being. You may have difficulty in shedding the last few pounds and will have to consider whether an increase in exercise intensity or a longer dieting period is worthwhile.

On reflection you may find that you are content with what you have achieved. If you have attained a weight within the BMI range for your height and are steadily following sensible eating and exercise principles, you should be more than satisfied with the results.

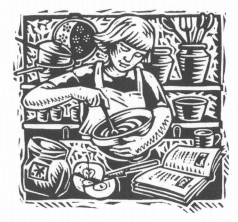

CHAPTER 9

RECIPES FOR WEIGHT CONTROL

This chapter offers a selection of delicious, low-fat calorie-controlled recipes that will appeal to both the weight watcher and the nondieter. Many of the dishes are ideal for entertaining as well as for family meals. Calorie and fat amounts per serving are given for each recipe. Check pages 66–67 for caloric values of any additional accompaniments. Ingredients are given in both metric and imperial measures, but they are not precise equivalents, so use either all-metric or all-imperial measures for any given recipe.

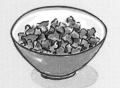

BREAKFASTS

If you are not a lover of breakfast, it can be tempting to cut out this first meal of the day. The advantages seem obvious: extra time in bed, a reduction in the total number of calories you eat each day, or being able to eat more at another mealtime. However, breakfast really is the most important meal.

Breakfast is exactly what the word implies— breaking a fast. By early morning it has usually been many hours since you ate anything, causing the sugar level in your blood to be very low. Food is needed to replenish the body's carbohydrate stores. If the level remains low, by midmorning you may be feeling faint, be unable to concentrate, and have an intense craving for food. This is when you will be tempted to reach for a snack, possibly a high-calorie convenience food like a doughnut or cookie.

Breakfast is the ideal time to eat foods that are rich in complex carbohydrates and protein to provide your body with energy for the day. The recipes and menu ideas that follow emphasize these two elements, and also supply fiber and plenty of the vitamins and minerals you need to get off to a good start.

All the family can sit down to the same breakfast, but those who are not watching their weight can eat more items and not necessarily low-calorie ones. This may involve buying a variety of cereals and a low-fat spread as well as butter. Children under five should always be given whole milk to drink and to have with cereal, while skim or low-fat milk can be used by the rest of the family to reduce their fat intake.

COMPLETE BREAKFAST IDEAS
If your breakfast supplies enough energy it should see you through until lunchtime. Each of the following menus provides a filling meal with which to start the day, and none is too high in calories.

MENU 1
Half a grapefruit provides at least 40 mg of vitamin C, which is more than half of an adult's daily requirement (60 mg) for this vitamin.

½ grapefruit
raisin porridge (see recipe, right)
tea/coffee (with skim milk or a slice of lemon)

210 cals, 3 g fat

MENU 2
Eggs, rich in protein, vitamins, and minerals, are also high in cholesterol. People with high cholesterol levels should limit them to four a week.

250 ml/9 fl oz orange juice
25 g/1 oz whole-wheat muesli with
low-fat (2%) milk
1 egg, scrambled, served with 1 slice of rye bread, toasted

398 cals, 15 g fat

MENU 3
If you prefer a cooked breakfast, fish provides a rich source of low-fat protein to set you up for the day.

115 g/4 oz white fish such as haddock, served with
1 tomato (grilled)
1 slice of whole-wheat bread
tea/coffee (with skim milk or a slice of lemon)

208 cals, 2.5 g fat

MENU 4
Yogurt is an excellent source of calcium, and strawberries provide a good amount of vitamin C.

muesli (see recipe, right)
225 g/8 oz low-fat plain yogurt with 3 strawberries (sliced)
tea/coffee (with skim milk or a slice of lemon)

443 cals, 12 g fat

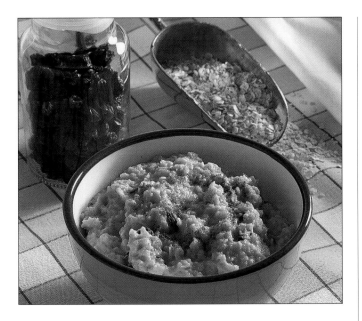

RAISIN PORRIDGE

177 cals, 2.5 g fat per serving

Serves 4

Oatmeal porridge can always be relied on to provide a warming start to the day, and it is an excellent source of soluble fiber.

300 ml/1¼ cups skim milk
600 ml/2½ cups water
55 g/2 oz (¼ cup) seedless raisins
large pinch cinnamon
160 g/5½ oz (2 cups) quick-cooking rolled oats

■ In a medium-size saucepan, bring the milk, water, raisins, and cinnamon to a boil. Stir in the oats, then reduce the heat and simmer for about 2 minutes or until the mixture thickens, stirring occasionally to prevent it from sticking to the pan.

DAILY MEAL PLAN

Breakfast: Menu 1 (page 132)
Mid-morning snack: Banana
Lunch: Crunchy Salad with Vinaigrette (page 139); 1 slice of whole-wheat pita bread; mineral water
Dinner: Stuffed Eggplants (page 147); 55 g/2 oz broccoli, 100 g/3½ oz carrots, and 150 g/5½ oz boiled new potatoes; 350 ml/12 fl oz fresh fruit juice
Dessert: Coeur à la Crème (page 156); herbal tea

Total for the day: 1406 calories, 31.5 g fat

As the total calories for the day are low, you could have a glass of wine or 300 ml/10 fl oz of beer with your dinner. This would add about 95 calories to the total.

HEALTHY EATING TIP
Nuts are highly nutritious. They are a rich source of vitamin E and also contain the B vitamins, thiamin and niacin. They are, however, high in fat, although it is mostly in the form of unsaturated fatty acids.

OAT, FRUIT, AND NUT MUESLI

304 cals, 10 g fat per serving

Serves 4

The fruits, nuts, and seeds in this recipe provide a range of nutrients, while the sugar in the fruit lends natural sweetness. You can store some of the muesli in an airtight container, if you do not need it right away.

115 g/4 oz mixed dried fruits such as raisins, cranberries, apricots, and prunes
55 g/2 oz mixed nuts and seeds such as walnuts and sunflower seeds
115 g/ 1½ cups quick-cooking rolled oats
2 pieces of fresh fruit such as apple, orange, peach, or nectarine

■ Cut up any large pieces of dried fruit and nuts. In a medium-size mixing bowl, stir together all the ingredients except the fresh fruit.
■ Prepare the fresh fruit as appropriate. For each serving, put one-quarter of the muesli in a bowl. Top with the fresh fruit and 1/2 cup low-fat (1%) milk or low-fat yogurt, as desired.

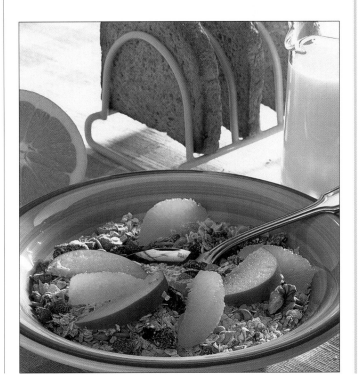

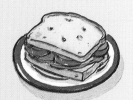

LIGHT MEALS AND SNACKS

When watching your weight it is often difficult to think of something both healthful and appealing to eat for a light meal or snack. It is all too easy to reach for convenience foods like cookies and chips—which are high in fat and calories and can ruin your weight-control plan.

Try some of the recipes on the following pages for low-fat alternatives. Several of the light meals can be turned into regular meals if desired. The salads can form light courses as they are, or be accompanied by low-fat cheese or cold meat. Additionally, they can be served as accompaniments to one of the main dishes given on pages 142 to 149. The Chinese Stir-Fried Vegetables on page 137 can also be enjoyed alongside a main course if calories allow. Salad dressings often add an unhealthy amount of fat to an otherwise healthy eating choice. Try the vinaigrette that goes with the crunchy salad on page 139, or concoct a low-fat dressing of your own, using nonfat yogurt, puréed tomatoes, or roasted red peppers for the base and adding fresh herbs and a flavored vinegar such as raspberry, tarragon, or sherry. When you do use an oil to make a dressing, try extra-virgin olive oil, hazelnut oil, or walnut oil. All are good choices because they have intense flavors and can be used effectively in small amounts.

If you don't have time to prepare one of these recipes, sandwiches are a practical healthy alternative. Be careful when buying ready-made sandwiches, as the fillings can often be high in fat. Avoid bacon, avocado, whole-milk cheese, and toppings such as coleslaw that have mayonnaise as a binding ingredient. If possible, make your own sandwiches (see page 128) and increase the ratio of bread to filling by slicing your bread thicker.

SHRIMP FAJITAS WITH SALSA

456 cals, 3 g fat per serving
Serves 4

Shrimps are a low-fat source of protein. Here, the traditional sour cream and guacamole have been replaced by coriander salsa and yogurt, which are lower in fat.

450 g/1 lb uncooked large shrimp, peeled and deveined
zest and juice of 1 lime
1 clove garlic, crushed
½ red chili, seeded and minced, or ¼ tsp crushed red pepper
1 tbsp freshly chopped coriander (cilantro)
¼ tsp salt plus freshly ground black pepper to taste
1 bunch green onions
12 soft flour tortillas
1 each red and yellow bell pepper, quartered and seeded
150 g/5½ oz (⅔ cup) low-fat plain yogurt

For the salsa
3 tbsp freshly chopped coriander (cilantro)
½ red chili, seeded and minced, or ¼ tsp crushed red pepper
zest and juice of 1 lime

- Preheat the oven to 180°C/350°F. Place the shrimp in a bowl with the lime zest and juice, garlic, chili, coriander, salt, and pepper and leave to marinate.
- For the salsa: finely chop two of the green onions; mix with the coriander, chili, and lime zest and juice. Season to taste.
- Wrap the tortillas in foil and warm in the oven for 15 minutes.
- Broil the peppers until the skins begin to char. Cool slightly; remove the skins and slice the peppers into strips. Cut the rest of the onions into slivers; arrange on a platter with the peppers.
- Heat a large nonstick skillet over high heat. Remove the shrimp from the marinade and put them in the skillet. Stir-fry until they turn pink and are cooked through.
- Spread some yogurt on a warm tortilla, add a few shrimp, top with the green onions, peppers, and salsa, and roll up.

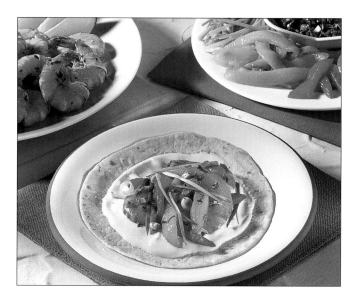

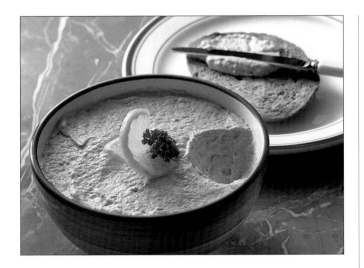

SMOKED MACKEREL PÂTÉ

332 cals, 22 g fat per serving

Serves 4

Oily fish is an important component of a balanced diet supplying valuable protein, calcium, vitamin D, and omega-3 fatty acids, all essential for good health.

275 g/9½ oz smoked mackerel, kippered herring,
    or other smoked fish
115 g/4 oz low-fat cream cheese
150 g/5½ oz (⅔ cup) low-fat plain yogurt
juice of half a lemon
2 tsp prepared horseradish
freshly ground black pepper to taste
4 slices of lemon and sprigs of parsley for garnish
4 slices of whole-wheat toast for serving

■ Carefully remove any bones from the mackerel, peel off the skin, then break the fish into small pieces.
■ Put all the ingredients in a blender or food processor and process until the mixture is thick and creamy. Press into a bowl or four small individual pots.
■ Chill until ready to serve. Garnish with lemon slices and sprigs of parsley and serve with slices of toast.

DAILY MEAL PLAN

Breakfast: Menu 3 (page 132)
Mid-morning snack: Whole-wheat roll with 55 g/2 oz cottage cheese
Lunch: Smoked Mackerel Pâté with toast; 360 ml/ 12 fl oz orange juice
Dinner: Chinese Chicken (page 148) with 150 g/5½ oz (¾ cup) boiled rice; glass of mineral water
Dessert: Melon Surprise (page 153); cup of herbal tea

Total for the day: 1,297 calories, 33.5 g fat

MEDITERRANEAN TOMATO SOUP

111 cals, 6.5 g fat per serving

Serves 4

Soup makes a filling meal and is nutritious because the cooking water retains some of the water-soluble vitamins from the vegetables. This low-calorie soup is also rich in potassium and beta-carotene.

900 g/2 lb (about 8) plum tomatoes
2 tbsp olive oil
1 small onion, chopped
½ large red bell pepper, seeded and chopped
1 clove garlic, crushed
2 tbsp red wine (optional)
2 tsp freshly chopped basil plus 4 sprigs for garnish
300 ml/1¼ cups hot chicken or vegetable stock
salt and freshly ground black pepper to taste

■ Place the tomatoes in a large bowl, pour boiling water over them, and leave them for a few moments. Remove from the boiling water with a slotted spoon and cool in a bowl of cold water for a few minutes. Peel off the skins and discard. Quarter the tomatoes and remove and discard the seeds.
■ Heat the oil in a large saucepan and lightly sauté the onion, bell pepper, and garlic. Add the tomatoes, red wine, and chopped basil. Bring this mixture to a boil and simmer gently for about 15 minutes.
■ Transfer the mixture to a blender or food processor and process at top speed until the contents are very smooth. Return the soup to the pan and add the hot stock to thin it to the desired consistency. Season with salt and pepper to taste. Divide the soup equally among four serving bowls and serve piping hot, garnished with the sprigs of basil.

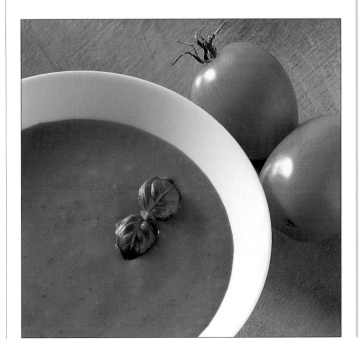

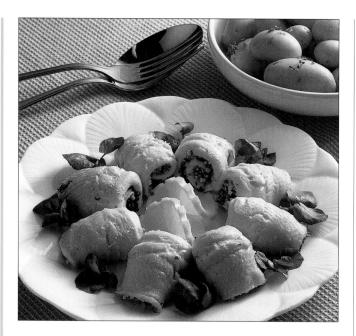

TROUT ROULADES WITH WATERCRESS AND MUSHROOM STUFFING

252 cals, 8.5 g fat per serving
Serves 4

This tasty, filling dish is incredibly low in calories, and yet its nutritional value is high, providing potassium and vitamins A, C, and D as well as protein.

15 g/1 tbsp low-fat margarine
4 green onions, finely chopped
75 g/2¾ oz (⅔ cup) chopped watercress
75 g/2¾ oz (1 cup) finely chopped mushrooms
75 g/2¾ oz (¾ cup) dry whole-wheat breadcrumbs
2 tbsp lemon juice
½ tsp salt plus freshly ground black pepper to taste
4 trout fillets each weighing about 150 g/5½ oz
4 lemon wedges and sprigs of parsley for garnish

■ Preheat the oven to 190°C/375°F. In a large nonstick skillet, heat the margarine until melted. Add the onions, watercress, and mushrooms and cook gently for about 5 minutes. Stir in the breadcrumbs and half the lemon juice and mix well. Season to taste then set aside while you prepare the fish.
■ Skin the fillets and lay them flat on a board with the skinned side uppermost. Cut each fillet in half lengthwise and sprinkle with the remaining lemon juice. Divide the stuffing into eight equal portions, placing it along the center of each fillet. Roll up each piece of fish from the tail end and secure firmly with a round toothpick. Place a large piece of foil on a baking sheet. Lightly grease the foil, place the fillets on top, then fold the foil over to seal as a parcel.
■ Bake for 20 to 25 minutes or until the fish is cooked through, and then remove the toothpicks. Arrange the stuffed fillets on a warm serving dish and garnish with the lemon wedges and parsley. Serve with boiled new potatoes.

FARFALLE WITH BROCCOLI AND FRESH TOMATOES

369 cals, 4 g fat per serving
Serves 2

This quick dish, which can be put together in just about the time it takes to boil the pasta, has fresh ingredients that are full of vitamins and flavor. It can be prepard even more quickly if you skip the step of peeling the tomatoes.

175 g/6 oz farfalle or other dried pasta
2 medium ripe plum tomatoes
1 tsp olive oil
1 red chili, seeded and minced, or ½ tsp crushed red pepper
1 clove garlic, crushed
175 g/6 oz broccoli, separated into florets
2 tbsp freshly chopped basil
½ tsp salt plus freshly ground black pepper to taste

■ Place the tomatoes in a large bowl, pour boiling water over them, and leave them for a few moments. Remove from the boiling water with a slotted spoon and cool in a bowl of cold water for a few minutes. Peel off the skins and discard. Quarter the tomatoes, remove and discard the seeds, and chop roughly.
■ Put the pasta to cook in plenty of boiling salted water.
■ In a small saucepan, gently infuse the oil with the chili and garlic over low heat. Do not allow to brown.
■ Blanch the broccoli florets in boiling salted water for 3 minutes, then drain.
■ Turn up the heat under the chili and garlic oil, add the basil, tomatoes, and seasoning, and cook for 1 minute.
■ Drain the cooked pasta and mix it with the broccoli and tomato mixture and serve in deep bowls. For a main course, increase the quantity of pasta to 225 g/8 oz and serve with a fresh green salad.

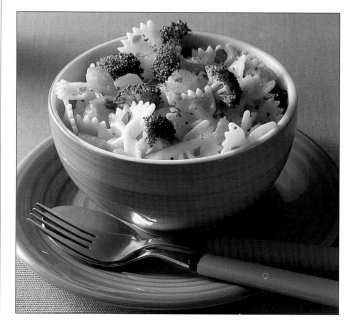

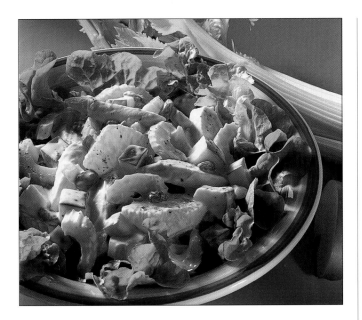

CHICKEN AND CELERY SALAD

287 cals, 6.5 g fat per serving
Serves 4

Lean chicken is an excellent source of protein, vitamins, and minerals. Here, it is combined with a mixture of fruit and vegetables for extra nutritional value.

450 g/1 lb cooked boneless chicken breasts
8 stalks celery, cut into bite-size pieces
2 red eating apples, such as McIntosh or red delicious
2 tbsp lemon juice
55 g/¹⁄₃ cup golden raisins
1 large grapefruit, peeled and segmented
300 g/10½ oz (1¼ cups) low-fat plain yogurt
salt and freshly ground black pepper to taste
1 small head of lettuce, divided into leaves

■ Remove and discard skin from the chicken and cut into thick strips. In a large bowl, mix the chicken and celery. Core and dice the apples, place them in another small bowl and sprinkle with the lemon juice to prevent them from discoloring.
■ Add the raisins and grapefruit segments to the chicken and celery, followed by the apple and lemon juice. Stir all the ingredients together well. Sir in the yogurt. Season to taste with the salt and pepper.
■ Arrange the lettuce leaves on a serving dish, pile the chicken mixture on top, and refrigerate until ready to serve.

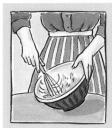

HEALTHY EATING TIP
Much of the fat content of chicken comes from the skin, so always remove it. Use breast meat whenever possible, as it is lower in fat than the thighs and drumsticks.

CHINESE STIR-FRIED VEGETABLES

188.5 cals, 11.5 g fat per serving
Serves 4

Whatever your diet restrictions, fresh vegetables can always be eaten in unlimited amounts, providing essential vitamins, minerals, and dietary fiber.

55 g/2 oz whole almonds
115 g/4 oz cauliflower, broken into florets
1 tbsp sunflower oil or vegetable oil
2 stalks celery, thinly sliced
4 green onions, thinly sliced
1 medium red bell pepper, seeded and cut into thin strips
115 g/4 oz button mushrooms, sliced
115 g/4 oz snow peas, trimmed
1 tsp grated fresh ginger, or ½ tsp dried ginger
2 cloves garlic, crushed
300 ml/1¼ cups vegetable stock
1 tsp sesame oil
2 tbsp soy sauce
2 tsp dry sherry (optional)
1 tbsp cornstarch
115 g/4 oz mung bean sprouts
coriander (cilantro) sprigs for garnish

■ Lightly toast the almonds. Blanch the cauliflower by dropping it into boiling water, cooking for 1 minute, then draining it. In a wok or large deep skillet, heat the oil over high heat. Add the celery, green onions, bell pepper, mushrooms, snow peas, ginger, and garlic and stir-fry, tossing the vegetables until they are just becoming tender.
■ Add the stock, sesame oil, soy sauce, and sherry if desired. Continue to toss the ingredients until the liquid boils. In a cup, blend the cornstarch with 2 tbsp of cold water. Add this to the wok and stir until the mixture thickens. Add the cauliflower, bean sprouts, and almonds. Heat thoroughly and serve immediately, garnished with coriander sprigs.

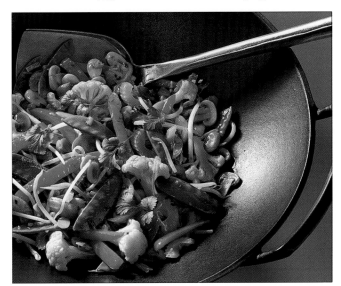

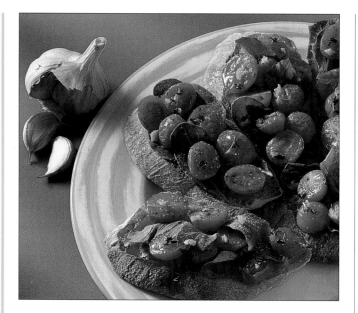

BRUSCHETTA WITH GRILLED TOMATOES AND ARUGULA

231 cals, 3 g fat per serving
Serves 2

The Mediterranean diet is recognized as both healthy and flavorful. Freshness of the ingredients is a major factor in the flavor. Here, broiling the tomatoes brings out their natural sweetness.

225 g/8 oz (16) ripe cherry tomatoes, halved
salt and freshly ground black pepper to taste
2 cloves garlic
2 tsp freshly chopped thyme
4 slices ciabatta bread
25 g/1 oz arugula (rocket) leaves

■ Place the halved tomatoes on a nonstick baking sheet and sprinkle lightly with salt and pepper.
■ Finely chop one garlic clove and scatter it over the tomatoes along with the thyme. Place under a preheated broiler and cook for 5 minutes until the tomatoes have softened and are slightly charred around the edges.
■ Cut the remaining garlic clove in half lengthwise. Toast the ciabatta slices and then rub them with the cut sides of garlic. Pile on the arugula leaves and cooked tomatoes and serve immediately.

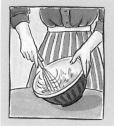

HEALTHY EATING TIP
Eating tomatoes regularly may reduce the risk of prostate cancer. Some researchers believe that the protective agents are lycopenes—bioflavonoids closely related to beta carotene.

SAFFRON COUSCOUS SALAD WITH SMOKED TROUT

226 cals, 3 g fat per serving
Serves 4

This salad is colorful and easy to make. It is high in protein and low in fat, having yogurt as a healthy alternative to an oil-based dressing.

225 g/8 oz couscous
1 tsp ground cumin
½ tsp ground coriander
¼ tsp salt plus freshly ground black pepper to taste
420 ml/1¾ cups vegetable stock
3 good pinches saffron
juice of 1 lemon
3 tbsp chopped fresh flat-leaf parsley
½ cucumber, diced
225 g/8 oz (16) cherry tomatoes, quartered
1 small bulb fennel, trimmed and diced
1 large carrot, peeled and diced (1 cup)
4 green onions, finely sliced
2 smoked trout fillets, approximately 150 g/5½ oz total
3 tbsp low-fat plain yogurt
3 tbsp chopped fresh mint
pinch of cayenne pepper

■ Put the couscous in a large heatproof bowl and stir in the cumin, coriander, and seasoning. In a small saucepan, bring the stock to a boil over high heat; stir in the saffron and lemon juice, then pour the stock over the couscous and mix well. Leave until the liquid has been absorbed, 10 to 15 minutes.
■ Fluff and loosen the couscous with a fork. Mix in the parsley and check for seasoning. Transfer to a glass salad bowl.
■ Scatter the vegetables over the couscous and flake the trout fillets over the top.
■ To make the dressing, mix together the yogurt and mint with a pinch of cayenne and a little salt. Serve separately.

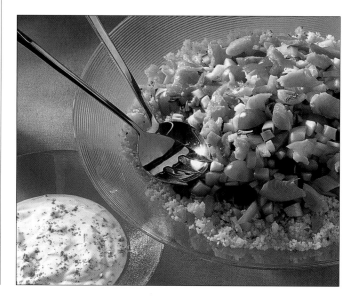

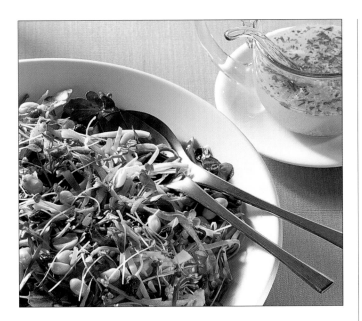

CRUNCHY SALAD WITH VINAIGRETTE

253 cals, 13 g fat per serving
Serves 4

Raw cabbage forms the crunchy base of this salad. It contains more micronutrients than lettuce, is a good source of vitamin C, and is high in dietary fiber.

½ small white cabbage
½ small red cabbage
1 bunch watercress
2 medium carrots
1 to 2 oz alfalfa sprouts (optional)
4 tbsp raisins
4 tbsp unsalted peanuts
2 tbsp lemon juice

For the vinaigrette:
80 ml/⅓ cup white wine vinegar
80 ml/⅓ cup lemon juice
2 tbsp olive oil
2 tsp whole-grain mustard
2 tsp honey
1 clove garlic, crushed (optional)
2 tbsp chopped fresh parsley
¼ tsp salt plus freshly ground black pepper to taste

■ To make the salad: wash and trim all the vegetables. Finely shred the white and red cabbages, remove the thick stems from the watercress, and coarsely grate the carrots. Place all the ingredients in a large salad bowl and toss to mix well.
■ To make the vinaigrette: put the vinegar, lemon juice, olive oil, mustard, honey, garlic, and parsley in a screw-top jar with a tight-fitting lid and shake to mix well. Add the salt and pepper to taste. Serve separately.

STUFFED BAKED POTATO

144 to 242 cals, 1 to 10 g fat per serving
Serves 1

Baked potatoes are packed with complex carbohydrates and are a great low-fat source of fiber and nutrients.

1 medium russet or baking potato (about 175g/6 oz)

■ Preheat oven to 220°C/425°F. Scrub the potato lightly and dry with a paper towel. Prick in several places with a sharp pointed knife. Bake for 45 to 50 minutes or until tender.
■ Cut the cooked potato in half lengthwise. Scoop the inside into a bowl, taking care not to break the skin. Mix the potato with any of the suggested fillings and season to taste.
■ Pile the mixture back into the potato shell and serve.

FILLINGS
25 g/1 oz mushrooms, chopped and lightly sautéed
30 calories, 3 g fat per serving

1 scrambled egg and chopped fresh parsley
111 calories, 9.5 g fat per serving

110 g/4 oz spinach, chopped and cooked, and lots of pepper
13 calories, 0.5 g fat per serving

55 g/2 oz flaked canned salmon and a sliced tomato
86 calories, 4 g fat per serving

55 g/2 oz canned sardines and cucumber
110 calories, 7 g fat per serving

55 g/2 oz baked beans and 25 g/1 oz grated low-fat Cheddar
107 calories, 4 g fat per serving

25 g/1 oz shrimp and watercress
29 calories, 0.5 g fat per serving

25 g/1 oz chopped ham and 1 tbsp corn kernels
54 calories, 1.5 g fat per serving

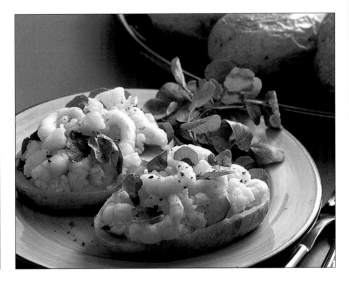

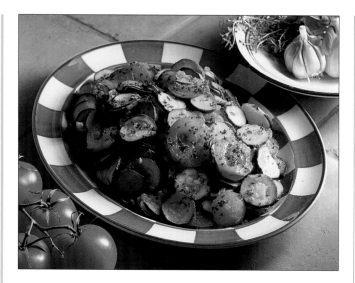

ZUCCHINI PROVENÇALE

64 cals, 1 g fat per serving

Serves 4

Zucchini are highly nutritious, containing good amounts of vitamin C, folate, and beta-carotene. Most of these nutrients are found in the tender, edible skin.

4 small zucchini, thinly sliced
2 small onions, thinly sliced
2 medium tomatoes, skinned and sliced
1 clove garlic, crushed
½ tsp salt plus freshly ground black pepper to taste
1 tbsp chopped fresh or 2 tsp dried basil or thyme
2 tbsp chopped fresh parsley for garnish

■ In a large saucepan, mix all the vegetables, the garlic, the seasoning, and basil or thyme. Bring to a simmer, cover, and cook gently until tender, 15 to 20 minutes. If the mixture seems to be a bit dry because the tomatoes were not very juicy, add a little chicken or vegetable stock.
■ Transfer to a warm serving dish, garnish with the parsley, and serve piping hot.

DAILY MEAL PLAN

BREAKFAST: Menu 2 (page 132)
MID-MORNING SNACK: 100 g/3½ oz fresh strawberries with 100 g/3½ oz low-fat plain yogurt
LUNCH: Zucchini Provençale with 2 slices of whole-wheat bread; glass of mineral water
DINNER: Jambalaya (page 149); 8-oz glass of fruit juice
DESSERT: Baked Stuffed Apples with Homemade Custard (page 155); cup of herbal tea

TOTAL FOR THE DAY: 1,487 calories, 33 g fat

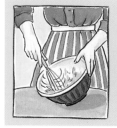

HEALTHY EATING TIP
Eggs are rich in protein, vitamins, and minerals. They are best stored in the main part of the refrigerator, instead of the door compartment, where they will keep for about three weeks.

SCRAMBLED EGGS WITH SMOKED SALMON AND COTTAGE CHEESE

361 cals, 15.5 g fat per serving

Serves 1

This is a quick lunch dish with a touch of luxury— delicious slivers of smoked salmon. The scrambled eggs are extra creamy, with the addition of low-fat cottage cheese. For toast, use a bread made with mixed grains and seeds. The crunchy texture makes all the difference.

2 small slices of mixed-grain bread
2 medium eggs
freshly ground black pepper to taste
2 tbsp low-fat cottage cheese
40 g/1½ oz smoked salmon, cut in thin strips
sprigs of fresh chives to garnish

■ Toast the bread and keep warm.
■ In a small bowl, beat the eggs with a little pepper. Heat a small nonstick skillet over medium heat and add the eggs. Cook, stirring continuously.
■ When the eggs are nearly cooked, stir in the cottage cheese and mix well. Add the smoked salmon and spoon immediately onto the toast. Garnish with chives.

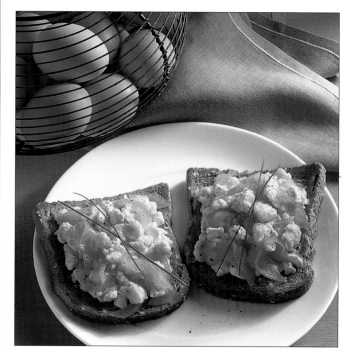

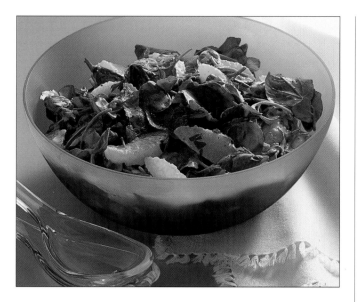

WATERCRESS AND ORANGE SALAD

90 cals, 3.5 g fat per serving

Serves 4

*Both the watercress and oranges in this colorful
and refreshing dish provide vitamins C and A.*

1 bunch watercress
2 large oranges
12 freshly shelled hazelnuts, if available, or
    2 tbsp chopped hazelnuts
150 g/5½ oz (⅔ cup) low-fat plain yogurt

For the dressing:
1 clove garlic, crushed
1 tbsp chopped fresh parsley
salt and freshly ground black pepper to taste

■ Remove any very thick stems from the watercress and
separate it into sprigs. Wash thoroughly and spin dry or dry
with paper towels. Peel the oranges and cut into segments,
making sure all the membranes and pith are removed. Do this
over a bowl so that all the juice is saved. Cut the segments in
half if they are large. In a serving bowl, toss together the
watercress, orange segments, and nuts.
■ In a small bowl, make the dressing: beat the reserved orange
juice, yogurt, garlic, and parsley and add the seasonings. Pour
the dressing over the salad and toss well. Let stand for about
20 minutes before serving to allow the flavors to blend.

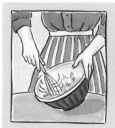

HEALTHY EATING TIP
Both watercress and oranges are
good sources of vitamins C and A.
These are antioxidants that can help
protect the body against infections
and some kinds of cancer.

CURRIED CHICKEN IN PITAS WITH A COOL RELISH

447 cals, 8 g per serving

Serves 4

*Spicy chicken stuffed into a pita makes a
fabulous yet healthy lunch. Tossing the chicken
in yogurt helps to tenderize the meat and
assist in the absorption of flavors.*

4 boneless, skinless chicken breasts, about 150 g/5½ oz each
2 tbsp curry paste or 1 tsp curry powder, or to taste
300 g/10½ oz (1¼ cups) low-fat plain yogurt
4 pita breads
wedges of lemon

For the relish:
1 small cucumber, diced
2 tbsp chopped fresh mint
¼ tsp salt plus freshly ground black pepper to taste

■ Cut each chicken breast into 5 or 6 even-sized chunks.
Blend the curry paste with ¼ cup of the yogurt and toss
the chicken in the mixture until it is well coated. Leave to
marinate for at least 15 minutes, or longer if possible.
■ To make the relish: stir the cucumber, mint, salt, and pepper
into the remaining 1 cup of yogurt. Chill until ready to serve.
■ Preheat a barbecue grill or broiler and soak 4 wooden skewers in water for 15 minutes to prevent them from burning.
■ Thread the chicken onto the skewers and season. Cook on a
rack over a barbecue or under a broiler for 10 to 15 minutes
or until the chicken is cooked through and beginning to char
at the edges.
■ Meanwhile, warm the pita breads and split them open.
Fill with the yogurt relish and the chicken. Serve with lemon
wedges to squeeze over the chicken.

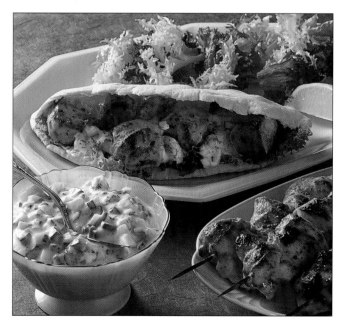

141

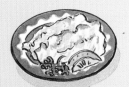

MAIN COURSES

Following a diet plan should not mean severely limiting your food selection or restricting your social life. These recipes, adaptations of popular dishes from home and abroad, meet low-fat dietary guidelines, and many are suitable for entertaining as well. Family members who are not watching their weight can have larger portions and eat more accompaniments to satisfy their needs, while toddlers can enjoy the same foods in smaller quantities or with slight adaptations.

The cooking methods are a significant aspect of low-fat dishes. For example, you can brown stew meat and roasts in a nonstick pan without the need for added fat. Cooking ground meat in the same way and then draining it will remove about 40 percent of the fat. Instead of brushing meat with oil, while broiling or grilling, marinate it beforehand. This will make it more tender and flavorful as well as prevent it from drying out. When roasting meat or poultry, place it on a rack in the roasting pan, so that the fat drains away from the meat. Leaving the skin on chicken helps to keep it moist while it cooks, but you can reduce the fat level significantly if you remove the skin before serving.

When preparing casseroles, you can make them healthier by using less meat and increasing the quantity of vegetables or adding dried legumes such as lentils. Soften onions in a little stock, wine, or water rather than in oil. Reduce the fat level even further by making the casserole in advance, then chilling it so that the fat will set on the surface and can be removed with a spoon.

RED PEPPER AND BASIL FRITTATA

182 cals, 7.5 g fat per serving
Serves 6

Frittata makes a delicious dish, eaten hot or cold, and this one is packed with vitamin C. The fat-free method used here for cooking onions down to a sweet, melting mass is useful for other recipes, particularly casseroles.

2 medium onions, thinly sliced
420 ml/1¾ cups vegetable stock
2 medium red bell peppers, quartered and seeded
3 medium potatoes, peeled, cut in 1.25-cm/½-in cubes
6 large eggs
½ tsp salt plus freshly ground black pepper to taste
15 g/½ oz fresh basil, shredded
1 tsp olive oil

- Heat a large nonstick skillet over moderate heat and add the onions. Allow them to color and soften slightly, then pour in 300 ml/1¼ cups of the stock. Cook, stirring occasionally, until the liquid has evaporated.
- Meanwhile, grill or broil the bell peppers until the skins are charred. Allow them to cool, then peel off and discard the skins and cut the peppers into thin strips. Cook the cubed potatoes in salted water for about 8 minutes or until tender. Drain and set aside.
- When the onion liquid has disappeared and the onions have browned a little, add half the remaining stock and allow it to bubble away and the onions to brown more. Repeat with the last of the stock. Remove onions to a plate and rinse the pan.
- In a large bowl, beat the eggs well, season with the salt and pepper, then add the basil, peppers, potatoes, and onions.
- Preheat the broiler. Heat the oil in the skillet and pour in the egg mixture. Cook over low heat for 10 minutes or until the underside is golden and the frittata is almost set. Set the skillet under the broiler until the top is set and golden. Let it stand for 5 minutes. Turn out and serve with a green salad.

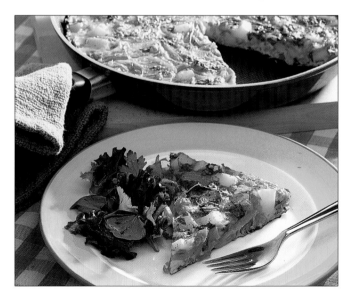

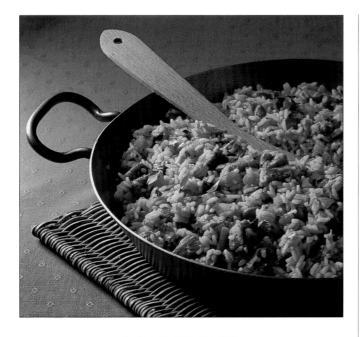

PORK PAELLA

434 cals, 12 g fat per serving

Serves 4

Traditionally, Spanish paella is made with seafood, chicken, and sausage, but for a healthy change this recipe calls for lean pork. It has only slightly more fat than skinless chicken and is a good source of protein, zinc, and B vitamins, especially B$_{12}$.

1 tbsp corn oil
450 g/1 lb tenderloin of pork, cut into 1.25-cm/½-in cubes
1 large onion, chopped
2 cloves garlic, crushed
1 tsp paprika
½ tsp ground turmeric
400 g/14 oz canned tomatoes, chopped, with their juice
360 ml/1½ cups chicken or vegetable stock
170 g/6 oz (1 cup) long-grain white rice
½ tsp salt plus freshly ground black pepper to taste
1 tbsp chopped fresh parsley for garnish

▪ In a nonstick wok or large, deep skillet with a lid, heat the oil over high heat. Add the pork and stir-fry until browned. Add the onion, garlic, paprika, and turmeric and cook for a few minutes more. Add the tomatoes, stock, and rice.
▪ Cover and simmer for 20 minutes or until the rice is cooked and all the liquid is absorbed. Stir occasionally and check that the mixture is not too dry (if it is, add a little more liquid). Season with the salt and pepper and garnish with the chopped parsley. Leave to stand for 5 minutes before serving.

MOROCCAN CHICKEN TAGINE WITH APRICOTS

335 cals, 9 g fat per serving

Serves 4

This fragrant stew features many of the flavors of Middle Eastern cookery, where the combination of meat and fruit in one dish is common.

1 whole chicken (approximately 1.3 kg/3 lb), jointed into
    8 pieces and skin removed, or 8 thighs and drumsticks
2 medium onions, finely chopped
2 cloves garlic, crushed
1 tbsp grated fresh ginger, or 1 tsp ground ginger
pinch of saffron
¼ tsp ground turmeric
2 tsp ground cumin
2 tsp ground coriander
1 tsp ground cinnamon
½ tsp each salt and ground black pepper
juice of 1 lemon
400 g/14 oz canned chickpeas, rinsed and drained
115 g/4 oz dried apricots
2 tbsp chopped fresh coriander leaves (cilantro) for garnish

▪ In a tagine or flameproof casserole, mix together the chicken, onion, garlic, fresh ginger, saffron, ground spices, salt, and pepper. Pour in the lemon juice, then add enough cold water to just cover. Bring to a simmer, cover, and cook very gently for 45 minutes.
▪ Stir the drained chickpeas and apricots into the casserole and simmer, uncovered, for 30 minutes more.
▪ Using a slotted spoon, transfer the chicken, chickpeas, and apricots to a warm serving dish. Return the casserole to the burner, set on high, and boil the liquid to reduce it by about one-third. Pour the sauce over the chicken and scatter the coriander on top before serving. Serve with plenty of couscous or rice to soak up the delicious sauce.

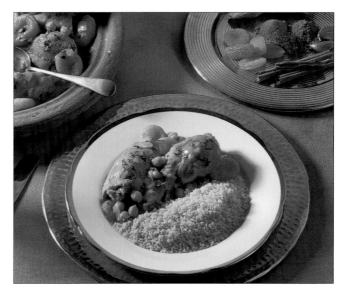

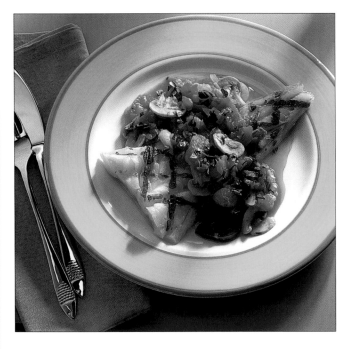

FISH CREOLE

198 cals, 4.5 g fat per serving

Serves 4

White fish such as cod or haddock is perfect for a dieter's menu. It is low in fat and high in protein.

1 medium onion, chopped
1 stalk celery, chopped
115 g/4 oz mushrooms, sliced
1 small green bell pepper, seeded and sliced
4 cloves garlic, minced
400 g/14 oz canned chopped tomatoes, with their juice
3 tbsp tomato purée
½ tsp salt plus freshly ground black pepper to taste
pinch of chili powder
dash of Tabasco sauce
1 tbsp olive oil
675 g/1½ lb cod or haddock fillets, skinned and cut
   into 4 pieces
1 tbsp chopped fresh parsley for garnish

■ In a large nonstick skillet over low heat, cook the onion, celery, mushrooms, bell pepper, and garlic for 10 minutes. Add the tomatoes, tomato purée, salt, pepper, chili powder, and Tabasco sauce. Simmer, uncovered, for 30 minutes or until the vegetables are tender and the sauce has thickened.
■ Heat the oil in a ridged grill pan or large skillet until slightly smoky. Place the fish in the pan and grill for 8 to 10 minutes, turning it once halfway through the cooking time (the fish should show grill marks from the pan). Pour the sauce over the fish and garnish with the parsley. Serve with steamed rice.

WARM TERIYAKI CHICKEN WITH SESAME DRESSING

284 cals, 8 g fat per serving

Serves 4

The tangy marinade in this recipe keeps the meat moist and adds flavor. The vegetables are cooked only briefly, so that they retain much of their vitamin content.

¼ cup teriyaki sauce
1 tbsp clear honey
½ tsp Chinese five spice powder (optional)
4 boneless, skinless chicken breasts, about 150 g/5½ oz each
225 g/8 oz green beans, trimmed
225 g/8 oz sugar snap peas, trimmed
225 g/8 oz broccoli florets

For the dressing:
1 tbsp soy sauce
1 tbsp clear honey
½ tsp sesame oil
1 tbsp sesame seeds, toasted and crushed
1 red chili, seeded and minced, or ½ tsp crushed red pepper
6 green onions, sliced

■ To make the marinade: mix together the teriyaki sauce, honey, and Chinese five spice powder. Put the chicken in a shallow dish and pour the marinade over it. Cover and marinate for at least 30 minutes, turning occasionally.
■ Remove the chicken from the marinade and cook under a preheated broiler for 15 minutes or until cooked through, basting occasionally with the marinade to give a glossy finish.
■ Meanwhile, cook the green beans, sugar snap peas, and broccoli florets in boiling salted water for 3 minutes.
■ For the dressing: whisk the soy sauce, honey, and sesame oil together. Mix in the sesame seeds, chili, and green onions.
■ Drain the vegetables, toss them in the dressing, and arrange on plates. Slice the chicken and place on top of the vegetables. Serve with boiled rice or rice noodles.

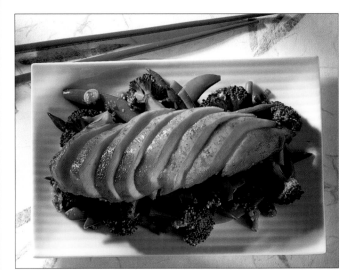

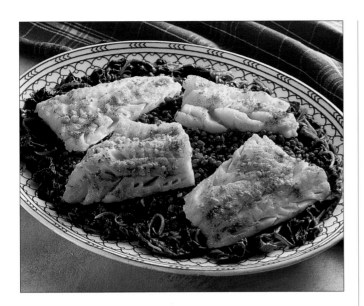

SPICED COD WITH LENTILS

342 cals, 5.5 g fat per serving

Serves 4

All legumes are a good, economical source of protein and also make fine thickeners for soups and stews. Lentils hold their texture and absorb flavors well.

225 g/8 oz lentils
2 tsp each ground cumin and coriander seeds
360 to 420 ml/1½ to 1¾ cups vegetable stock
salt and freshly ground black pepper to taste
½ tsp Chinese five spice powder (optional)
2.5-cm/1-in piece fresh ginger, grated
grated zest and juice of 1 lime
4 pieces cod fillet, each about 150 g/5½ oz, skinned
1 clove garlic, crushed
1 tsp olive oil
450 g/1 lb young leaf spinach

■ In a large saucepan, stir together the lentils, half of the cumin and coriander, and 360 ml/1½ cups of the stock. Season with pepper, but no salt, as it keeps lentils from cooking properly. Simmer, covered, for 30 to 45 minutes or until the liquid is absorbed and the lentils are tender. Check the lentils half way through the cooking time, adding more stock if needed.
■ Mix the remaining spices with the five-spice powder, ginger, lime zest, half of the lime juice, and a little salt and pepper. Rub this paste into the cod fillets. Set aside.
■ When the lentils are almost cooked, place the cod fillets on a lightly oiled baking sheet and broil about 10 cm/4 in from the heat for 5 to 7 minutes, depending on thickness.
■ Meanwhile, in a large skillet, sauté the garlic in the olive oil. Gradually add the spinach, tossing it as it comes into contact with the heat, until it has just wilted. Season with salt and pepper. Stir the remaining lime juice into the lentils and check the seasoning.
■ Serve the cod on a bed of the spinach and lentils.

COUNTRY CASSEROLE

233 cals, 8 g fat per serving

Serves 4

Light ale adds wonderful flavor to this dish and only 24 calories per portion. You could substitute beer for similar results.

1 tbsp olive oil
450 g/1 lb lean beef round, cut into 1-inch cubes
1 medium onion, sliced
2 large carrots, sliced
1 clove garlic, crushed (optional)
115 g/4 oz mushrooms, wiped and sliced
300 ml/1¼ cups light ale or beer
1 cube beef bouillon
1 tsp vinegar
1 tsp brown sugar
1 bay leaf
1 tbsp cornstarch
salt and freshly ground black pepper to taste
1 tbsp chopped fresh parsley for garnish

■ Preheat the oven to 180°C/350°F. In a medium-size nonstick skillet, heat the oil over high heat and brown the meat on all sides. Transfer the meat to a 1.75 liter/2-quart casserole. Add the onion, carrots, garlic, and mushrooms.
■ In a measuring cup, blend the ale, beef bouillon cube, vinegar, and brown sugar. Pour this mixture over the meat and vegetables and add the bay leaf. Cover and cook in the oven for 1½ to 2 hours or until the meat is tender.
■ In a cup, blend the cornstarch with 1 tbsp water, and then stir the mixture into the casserole. Return to the oven for 15 minutes more to allow the gravy to thicken. Season to taste.
■ Serve piping hot, garnished with the chopped parsley and accompanied by steamed green beans and boiled potatoes.

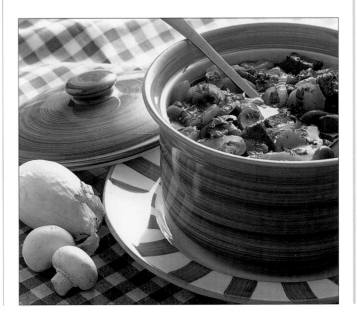

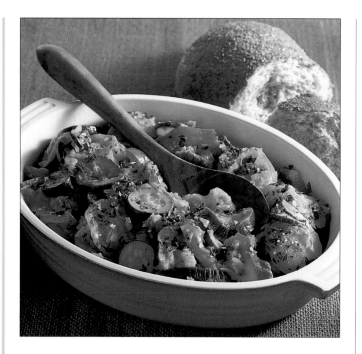

RATATOUILLE

110 cals, 4 g fat per serving
Serves 4

A dish that combines a variety of vegetables helps ensure a balanced diet. This recipe offers a range of nutrients and is particularly rich in vitamin A.

1 medium eggplant, about 350 g/12 oz, sliced 2.5 cm/1 in thick
2 small zucchini, about 225 g/8 oz, sliced 2.5 cm/1 in thick
1 tbsp olive oil
2 small onions, chopped
2 cloves garlic, crushed
1 medium red bell pepper, seeded and sliced into rings
1 medium green bell pepper, seeded and sliced into rings
2 tbsp chopped fresh parsley
2 medium tomatoes, skinned and sliced
salt and freshly ground black pepper

■ Place the eggplant and zucchini in a colander, sprinkle with salt, and press down with a plate; place heavy weights on top to hold in place. Leave for an hour and then rinse and pat dry with paper towels. While this step is not essential, the flavor of the dish will be greatly enhanced by it.
■ In a large, deep skillet, heat the oil over low heat; add the onion and garlic and cook for about 5 minutes. Add the peppers, eggplant, zucchini, and half of the parsley. Cover the skillet and simmer gently for 35 minutes or until the vegetables are soft but retain their shapes.
■ Stir in the tomato slices gently, keeping the various foods intact, and simmer for about 10 minutes more with the lid off, so that the tomato is heated through and the liquid reduced. Season with salt and pepper if necessary.
■ Transfer to a warm serving dish and sprinkle with the remaining parsley before serving.

FISH KEBABS WITH TARRAGON AND SESAME OIL SEASONING

140 cals, 4 g fat per serving
Serves 4

These kebabs made with chunks of cod provide a nutritious, low-calorie meal. For entertaining, in place of the cod you could use monkfish or shellfish such as shrimps or scallops.

450 g/1 lb thick cod fillet, skinned and cut into
    2.5-cm/1-in cubes
1 medium green bell pepper, seeded and cut into squares
    about 2.5 cm/1 in
4 firm small tomatoes, cut into quarters
12 button mushrooms, wiped clean
8 bay leaves
16 seedless grapes
1 tbsp sesame oil for brushing
fresh lemon juice
2 tsp chopped fresh tarragon or 1 tsp dried tarragon

■ On a board, divide all the ingredients, except the oil, lemon juice, and tarragon, into four equal piles. To make the kebabs, thread the fish cubes and different vegetable and fruit items in turn onto eight lightly greased skewers.
■ Preheat the broiler. Brush the kebabs with some of the sesame oil. Sprinkle with plenty of lemon juice and tarragon.
■ Lay the kebabs on a baking sheet. Broil about 6 inches from the heat for 15 to 20 minutes, turning frequently, until the fish and vegetables are cooked. Brush with the remaining oil and sprinkle with more lemon juice and tarragon each time you turn them.
■ Serve accompanied by steamed green vegetables in season or a salad and boiled potatoes or rice.

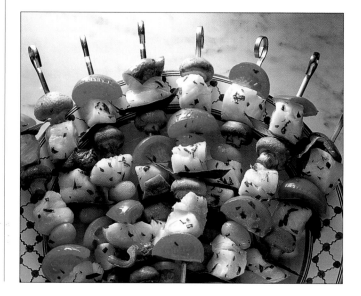

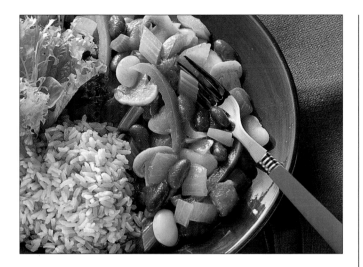

MIXED BEAN GOULASH

242 cals, 4.5 g fat per serving
Serves 4

For people who are eating less meat or none, this hearty goulash is an excellent source of complete protein.

115 g/4 oz dried butter beans
115 g/4 oz dried red kidney beans
1 tbsp corn oil
2 medium onions, chopped
2 stalks celery, chopped
115 g/4 oz mushrooms, wiped and sliced
1 medium green bell pepper, seeded and sliced
1 tbsp paprika
400 g/14 oz canned tomatoes, chopped, with their juice
1/2 tsp salt plus freshly ground black pepper to taste

■ Soak both types of beans in a large bowl of cold water for 8 to 10 hours. Drain them, transfer to a large saucepan, and cover with fresh cold water. Bring to a boil and boil rapidly for 10 minutes, skimming any foam from the surface. Lower the heat, cover, and simmer for 40 minutes or until tender.
■ Meanwhile, in a large flameproof casserole, heat the oil over high heat and sauté the onion and celery for 3 minutes. Add the mushrooms and bell pepper and cook for 2 minutes more. Stir in the paprika, the tomatoes with their juice, seasonings, and 480 ml/2 cups water. Stir well and bring to a boil.
■ Drain the beans and add them to the casserole. Lower the heat, cover, and simmer for 30 minutes, stirring occasionally. Serve accompanied by brown rice and a green salad.

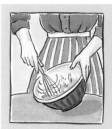

HEALTHY EATING TIP
Eaten with a grain food such as rice, kidney beans are a good source of fat-free protein. Red kidney beans are high in potassium and iron and also contain phosphorus, folate, and zinc.

STUFFED EGGPLANT

289 cals, 9.5 g fat per serving
Serves 4

Native to India, the eggplant has become a popular vegetable in the West and when baked is low in calories. The addition of other vegetables and rice to this recipe increases protein, carbohydrates, and fiber.

2 medium eggplants (900 g/2 lb), trimmed and cut in half lengthwise
2 tbsp corn oil
1 medium onion, finely chopped
1 stalk celery, finely chopped
1 large carrot, finely chopped
115 g/4 oz (2/3 cup) brown rice
2 cloves garlic, crushed (optional)
1/4 cup tomato purée
salt and freshly ground black pepper to taste
55 g/11/4 cups fresh breadcrumbs
1 tbsp chopped fresh herbs or 1 tsp dried herbs
55 g/2 oz (1/2 cup) shredded low-fat Cheddar cheese

■ Preheat the oven to 180°C/350°F. Scoop out the flesh of the eggplants, taking care not to break the shells, chop the flesh, and put the shells aside. In a large saucepan, heat the oil over high heat. Add the eggplant flesh, onion, celery, carrot, and rice and sauté for a few minutes, stirring well. Stir in half of the garlic, the tomato purée, and 360 ml/11/2 cups water.
■ Lower the heat, cover, and simmer for 40 minutes or until the rice and vegetables are cooked and the mixture has thickened. Season to taste with salt and pepper. Pile the mixture into the four eggplant shells.
■ Mix the breadcrumbs, herbs, and remaining crushed garlic and sprinkle over the filled shells. Place the shells on a baking sheet and bake for 15 minutes.
■ Sprinkle the cheese over the top of the eggplants and set them under a hot broiler until the cheese melts and begins to turn golden. Serve hot, accompanied by a green salad.

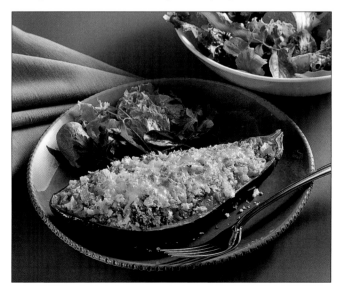

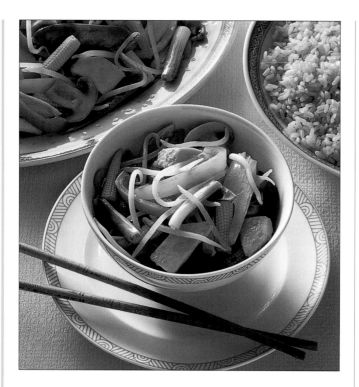

CHINESE CHICKEN

381 cals, 5.5 g per serving
Serves 4

The high protein and low-fat value of the chicken in this recipe is complemented by the vegetable mixture, which provides vitamins and other vital nutrients.

185 g/6 oz (1 cup) long-grain brown rice
225 g/8 oz cooked chicken, skin removed
1 tsp corn oil
1 tsp grated fresh ginger or ½ tsp ground ginger
1 clove garlic, crushed
1 each small red and yellow bell pepper, seeded and sliced
115 g/4 oz snow peas
115 g/4 oz canned baby corn
115 g/4 oz mushrooms, sliced
4 stalks celery, sliced
1 bunch green onions, sliced in 4-cm/1½-inch lengths
115 g/4 oz mung bean sprouts
2 tbsp soy sauce
¼ cup dry sherry (optional)
salt and freshly ground black pepper to taste

■ Put the rice on to cook. Cut the chicken into bite-size pieces. In a wok or large, deep skillet, heat the oil over high heat; add the ginger and garlic and stir-fry for 5 seconds. Add the bell peppers, snow peas, baby corn, mushrooms, and celery and stir-fry for 2 to 3 minutes more.
■ Add the chicken and cook for 2 minutes, then add the green onions, bean sprouts, soy sauce, and sherry and allow to bubble for about 1 minute. Season to taste.
■ Transfer to a warm serving dish and serve with the rice.

DEVILED LAMB

382 cals, 24 g fat per serving
Serves 4

Lamb is high in protein, rich in B vitamins, and is an excellent source of both zinc and iron. Choose cuts that are lean to keep the fat and calorie content low. By sautéing the lamb in a nonstick pan, you can seal in the juices without having to add oil to the recipe.

8 lamb neck cutlets or lean lamb loin chops,
    about 1 kg/2¼ lb total
2 stalks celery, sliced
1 medium onion, chopped
2 medium tomatoes, sliced
2 tsp dry mustard
150 ml/5 fl oz (⅔ cup) beef stock
150 ml/5 fl oz (⅔ cup) dry red wine or beef stock
1 tsp Worcestershire sauce
salt and freshly ground black pepper to taste

■ Trim any visible fat from the lamb. In a large, deep nonstick skillet over high heat, sauté the cutlets with the celery and onion until they are brown and the surface of the meat is sealed. Arrange the tomatoes over the meat.
■ Preheat the oven to 180°C/350°F. In a measuring cup, mix the mustard to a paste with a little of the stock, then blend in the rest of the stock, the red wine, and the Worcestershire sauce. Pour the mixture over the meat and bring to a boil.
■ Transfer the lamb and other ingredients to a large casserole, cover, and cook in the oven for approximately 1½ hours or until the meat is tender and beginning to come away from the bone. Season to taste.
■ Allow the casserole to cool completely, skim any fat that has risen to the surface, and then reheat.
■ Serve with mashed potatoes and fresh vegetables in season.

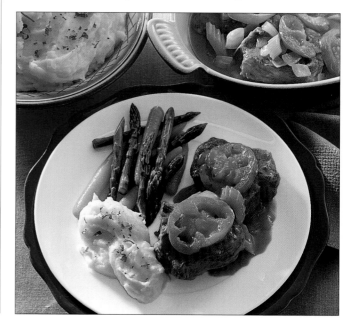

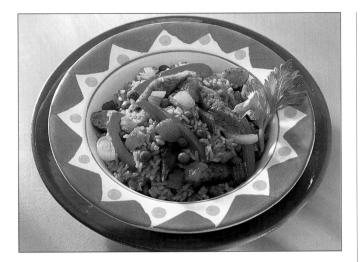

JAMBALAYA

448 cals, 14 g fat per serving
Serves 4

This spicy Spanish-Creole dish is rich in nutrients and fiber. Sausages are used for taste but to lower the fat content you could use skinless chicken instead.

1 tsp corn oil
1 medium onion, chopped
1 stalk celery, chopped
½ red bell pepper, seeded and cut into strips
1 clove garlic, chopped
1 tsp chili powder
225 g/8 oz (1⅓ cups) long-grain brown rice
480 ml/16 fl oz (2 cups) chicken stock
400 g/14 oz canned chopped tomatoes, with their juice
450 g/1 lb low-fat sausages, broiled and cut into chunks
75 g/2½ oz (½ cup) frozen peas
3 drops Tabasco sauce
salt and freshly ground black pepper

■ In a large skillet over high heat, sauté the onion, celery, and bell pepper for 5 minutes. Stir in the garlic, chili powder, and rice. Cook until the rice is opaque. Stir in the stock and tomatoes. Bring to a boil, lower the heat, and simmer for 30 to 35 minutes or until the rice is tender but still firm.
■ Add the sausage chunks to the pan along with the frozen peas and Tabasco sauce. Continue to cook for 10 minutes more or until the peas and sausage are heated through and the liquid is fully absorbed. Add salt and pepper to taste.

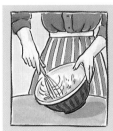

HEALTHY EATING TIP
As rice is gluten-free it is safe for people with wheat intolerance. Because brown rice goes through only minimal milling, it contains a greater amount of vitamins, minerals, and fiber than white rice.

SMOKED HADDOCK *EN PAPILLOTE* WITH TOMATO SALSA

156 cals, 1.5 g fat per serving
Serves 4

Baking en papillote *(in a paper parcel) keeps food moist, as all the juices are sealed in. The salsa here is a tasty fat-free alternative to traditional butter sauces.*

2 medium ripe tomatoes
½ medium red onion, finely chopped
½ medium red bell pepper, seeded and finely chopped
½ red chili, seeded and finely chopped, or ¼ tsp crushed red pepper
grated zest and juice of 1 lime
salt and freshly ground black pepper to taste
4 pieces of smoked haddock fillet, each about 150 g/5½ oz
115 g/4 oz asparagus tips, sugar snap peas, or green beans

■ For the salsa: place the tomatoes in a large bowl, pour boiling water over them, and leave for a few minutes. Remove from the boiling water with a slotted spoon and cool in a bowl of cold water for a few minutes. Peel off the skins and discard. On a chopping board, quarter the tomatoes; remove and discard the seeds, then chop finely. Mix with the onion, bell pepper, chili, and lime zest and juice. Season and set aside.
■ Meanwhile, preheat the oven to 220°C /425°F.
■ Cut out four 38-cm/15-in diameter circles of parchment paper or aluminum foil, fold in half to crease, and then open out. Brush lightly with a little oil. Place a piece of fish to one side of the crease on each paper circle. Spoon some salsa on top of the fish, and divide the asparagus tips among the parcels. Seal the parcels by pleating (folding) around the edges. Chill the remaining salsa.
■ Place the parcels on baking sheets and bake for 12 minutes.
■ Serve the parcels unopened, for your guests to fully savor the aroma as they tear open the paper. Serve the reserved salsa separately for a hot/cold contrast.

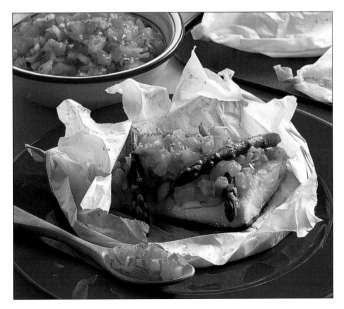

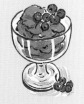

DESSERTS

Hidden fat and sugar in recipes and ready-made desserts can often be the downfall of a weight-management plan. But being on a diet doesn't mean you have to forgo desserts altogether. By making your own you can control your calorie and fat content.

Because it is completely fat-free, one of the most suitable foods for dessert is fresh fruit. Although most fruits are very sweet when ripe, the sugar content is from natural (intrinsic) sugars. Choose vine- or tree-ripened fruits that you can happily eat without added sugar. Be careful with canned fruits, as they are often preserved in calorie-laden syrup; look instead for those that are packed in their own juice. Topping your fruit with low-fat yogurt instead of cream or ice cream is an easy way to cut back on calories.

Flavored yogurt is a quick and nutritious dessert in its own right. The range available varies greatly in calorie and fat content, so check labels and try to find low-fat, low-sugar varieties.

This section gives you the opportunity to have dessert and still stick to a healthy and calorie-controlled diet. As you will see, most of the recipes contain less sugar than those in other recipe books (except for meringue). Adding dried fruit is one way to sweeten cakes and puddings so that they need no sugar, or at least require less than they would normally. The fruit increases the fiber content as well. Flavorings such as vanilla, cinnamon, cloves, grated fresh ginger, and orange zest heighten the sweetening effect.

EXOTIC FRUITS

Many exotic or unusual fruits are becoming more widely available and can add nutritious variety to your diet. The fruits described below can be served on their own as a dessert or added to a fruit salad.

PAPAYA

Cut in half from top to bottom and scoop out the seeds. Cut into slices like a melon and sprinkle with lemon juice, or cut into chunks and serve in a fruit salad.
Per 100 g: 36 calories, trace fat

PASSION FRUIT

Cut in half around the middle, scoop out the aromatic yellow, juicy pulp, and eat it with a teaspoon. The seeds are eaten, not discarded. It is delicious added to fruit punch and can also be used to add flavor to fruit pies.
Per 100 g: 36 calories, 0.5 g fat

LYCHEE (LITCHI NUT)

Serve as a dessert fruit on its own or add to fruit salad. Pinch the outer skin to crack it, then peel it off. Discard the stone. The flesh is white and juicy with a delicate flavor.
Per 100 g: 58 calories, trace fat

MANGO

Do not prepare until just before serving. Cut the fruit lengthwise, peel the skin back with a knife, and scoop out the pulp with a spoon. The orange/yellow flesh is very juicy and has a delicate fragrance and taste.
Per 100 g: 57 calories, trace fat

KIWI FRUIT

Cut in half around the middle and scoop out the pulp with a teaspoon in the same way you would eat a boiled egg. Alternatively, peel carefully and slice. Add to fruit salads or use to decorate puddings.
Per 100 g: 49 calories, 0.5 g fat

FIGS

Remove the stalk and slice in half lengthwise. The skin and flesh can be eaten as well as the seeds and sweet pulp.
Per 100 g: 43 calories, trace fat

GUAVA

Cut in half and scoop out the flesh with a teaspoon. The seeds should be eaten. Can be enjoyed raw or baked.
Per 100 g: 26 calories, 0.5 g fat

POMEGRANATE

Cut in half across the middle like a grapefruit and use a teaspoon to prise out the sections. Eat the seeds.
Per 100 g: 51 calories, trace fat

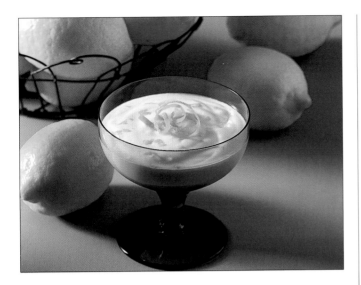

SYLLABUB

69 cals, 0.5 g fat per serving
Serves 4

This light and tangy dish is traditionally made with cream but yogurt makes a very healthy, low-fat alternative and adds protein and calcium to the diet.

1 unwaxed lemon
300 g/10½ oz (1¼ cups) low-fat plain yogurt
2 tbsp white wine
2 tbsp fresh lemon juice
honey to taste

■ Pare off a few fine strips of lemon zest and reserve to garnish the finished dish, then grate the rest. In a medium-size bowl, blend together the yogurt, wine, lemon juice, and grated rind and stir to form a smooth mixture.
■ Add honey to taste.
■ Spoon into four footed dessert dishes or wine glasses and chill for at least an hour. Garnish each syllabub with a little lemon zest just before serving.

DAILY MEAL PLAN

BREAKFAST: Oat, Fruit, and Nut Muesli (page 133); 330 ml/11 fl oz fresh orange juice
MID-MORNING SNACK: Nectarine
LUNCH: Shrimp Fajitas with Salsa (page 134); glass of mineral water
DINNER: Red Pepper and Basil Frittata (page 142) served with Crunchy Salad with Vinaigrette (page 139); glass of mineral water
DESSERT: Syllabub; herbal tea

TOTAL FOR THE DAY: 1519 calories, 38 g fat

SUMMER FRUIT ROULADE

189 cals, 5.5 g fat per serving
Serves 6

Summer berries are not only delicious but also rich in vitamin C. The yogurt adds a rich, creamy taste. For fewer calories, use a low-fat or nonfat type.

3 large eggs
85 g/3 oz (⅓ cup) granulated sugar
grated zest of 1 orange
85 g/3 oz (¾ cup plus 1 tbsp) all-purpose flour, sifted
pinch of salt
115 g/4 oz (½ cup) plain yogurt
350 g/12 oz mixed summer berries
confectioners sugar for dusting

■ Line a 20- x 30-cm/8- x 12-in jelly roll pan with baking parchment before you start to prepare the cake. Preheat the oven to 190°C/375°F.
■ In a large bowl, beat the eggs, sugar, and orange zest with an electric mixer set on medium, until the mixture is pale and mousse-like and the beaters leave a thick trail.
■ Sift the flour and salt over the mixture and quickly and carefully fold in, using a large rubber scraper. Be careful not to knock out too much air. Pour into the prepared pan and shake gently to distribute the batter evenly.
■ Bake on the center shelf of the oven for 12 to 15 minutes or until the sponge is golden and springy to the touch.
■ Remove from the oven and turn out onto a sheet of baking parchment. Carefully peel away the base paper, then start to roll up the roulade and fresh parchment from the short side. Leave to cool wrapped in the parchment.
■ When you are ready to serve the roulade, gently unroll the sponge, spread with the yogurt, and scatter the berries evenly over the top.
■ Roll up the roulade, lifting away the paper as you roll. Dust the roulade with a little confectioners sugar.

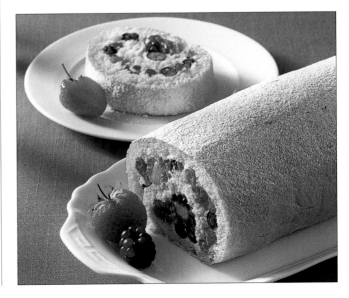

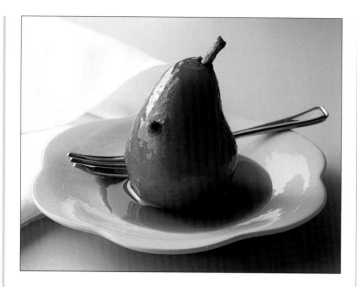

PEARS IN RED WINE

188 cals, trace fat per serving
Serves 4

Pears provide a useful source of fiber, vitamin C, and potassium. The addition of red wine or cider makes this a flavorful dessert.

4 large firm ripe pears
55 g/2 oz (¼ cup) granulated sugar
300 ml/10 fl oz (1¼ cups) red wine
1 tsp fresh lemon juice
2 cinnamon sticks
4 whole cloves
2 tsp cornstarch

■ Peel the pears, keeping them whole with stems attached. In a large saucepan bring the sugar, wine, lemon juice, and cinnamon sticks to a boil and cook until the liquid reduces a little.
■ Stick a clove in each pear, then place them in the wine mixture. Cover and simmer gently for 25 to 30 minutes or until the pears are just tender when tested with the tip of a sharp knife. Turn the pears once during cooking to ensure even coloring. Transfer the pears carefully with a slotted spoon to a large serving dish or four individual dishes.
■ Remove the cloves and cinnamon sticks. Boil the remaining liquid until it is reduced slightly. Blend the cornstarch with 1 tbsp cold water and add it to the syrup, stirring until it thickens. Pour the syrup over the pears. Serve them warm or chilled.

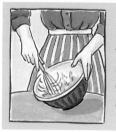

HEALTHY EATING TIP
If you would prefer to serve an alcohol-free dessert, use grape juice instead of red wine for the pears. This reduces the energy content as grape juice has about half the calories of red wine.

MIXED FRUIT FOOL

176 cals, 1 g fat per serving
Serves 4

Dried fruit is high in fiber and is a concentrated source of nutrients, especially iron and potassium. Use any mix that suits your taste, but don't include prunes in this dessert as they will discolor it.

225 g/8 oz mixed dried fruit such as peaches,
    apricots, pears, and apples
240 ml/1 cup tea made with 1 fruit-flavored or Earl Grey teabag
1 banana, peeled
juice of half a lemon
225 g/8 oz plain low-fat yogurt
few drops of almond extract to taste (optional)

■ From the mixed dried fruit, choose three apricots and set them aside. Place the remaining fruit in a medium-size bowl, cover with the tea, and soak for at least 12 hours to obtain maximum flavor.
■ Transfer the soaked fruit and liquid to a medium-size saucepan over low heat and simmer gently until tender, about 15 minutes. Drain the fruit well and place with the banana and lemon juice in a food processor or blender. Purée until smooth, then press through a sieve. Place the puréed fruit in a large bowl and fold in the yogurt. Taste for sweetness and add a few drops of almond extract if desired.
■ Divide equally among four dessert dishes or footed glasses. Chop the reserved apricots and use to garnish. Keep refrigerated until just before serving.

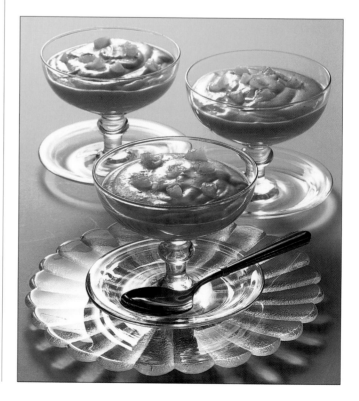

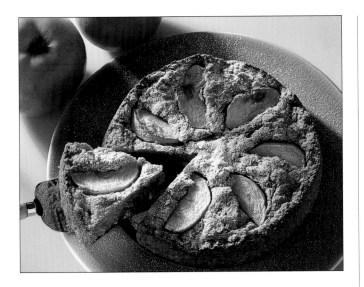

APPLE CAKE

267 cals, 12.5 g fat per serving

Serves 8

Cake is one food that dieters feel they should forgo, but here is a healthy alternative to high-calorie store-bought products.

225 g/8 oz (1¾ cups) whole-wheat flour, sifted
2 tsp baking powder
1 tsp ground cinnamon
1 tsp ground cloves
115 g/4 oz (1 stick) margarine
115 g/4 oz (½ cup) firmly packed brown sugar
3 medium cooking apples, peeled and cored

■ Preheat the oven to 190°C/375°F. In a medium-size mixing bowl, stir together the flour, baking powder, and spices, and then rub in the margarine until the mixture resembles bread-crumbs. Stir in the sugar. Put aside half an apple and grate the remaining ones. Stir them into the mixture.
■ Place the batter in a lightly greased 20-cm /8-in round cake pan. Cut the reserved apple into slender wedges and arrange on top. Bake for 35 minutes or until a knife inserted near the center comes out clean and the top is brown and crisp.

DAILY MEAL PLAN

BREAKFAST: *Menu 4 (page 132)*
MID-MORNING SNACK: *Orange*
LUNCH: *Scrambled Eggs with Smoked Salmon and Cottage Cheese (page 140); mineral water*
DINNER: *Warm Teriyaki Chicken with Sesame Dressing (page 144); green salad; glass of fresh fruit juice*
DESSERT: *Apple Cake; cup of herbal tea*

TOTAL FOR THE DAY: *1,760 calories, 61 g fat*

MELON SURPRISE

109 cals, 0.5 g fat per serving

Serves 4

This versatile fruit dish is low in calories and contains beta-carotene and vitamin C as well. The mixture of fruits ensures a variety of textures and colors that will delight both the palate and the eye.

4 small cantaloupe melons
1 pink grapefruit
1 large orange
1 kiwi fruit
115 g/4 oz white seedless grapes
a few strawberries and mint leaves to garnish

■ Carefully cut off the tops of the melons and keep them to one side. Scoop out the seeds with a teaspoon. Use a ball cutter to remove the melon flesh, taking care not to pierce the sides. Reserve the melon balls and juice in a large bowl.
■ Cut the grapefruit and orange into segments, taking care to remove all skin and pith. Cut the segments in half and add to the melon balls.
■ Peel the kiwi fruit, cut into slices, cut the slices in half and add with the grapes to the melon and citrus fruit.
■ Mix all the fruit together taking care not to break up the pieces. Chill the bowl of fruit in the refrigerator for at least an hour before serving.
■ Divide the fruit mixture equally among the four melon shells, which make attractive serving dishes, then pour the juices over, and decorate with one or two strawberries and mint leaves. Replace the reserved top of each melon just before serving.

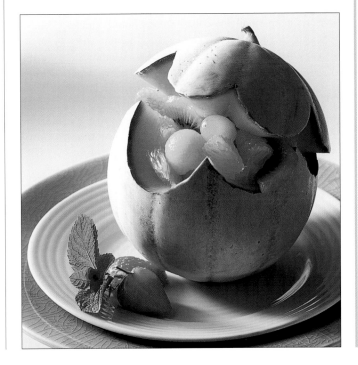

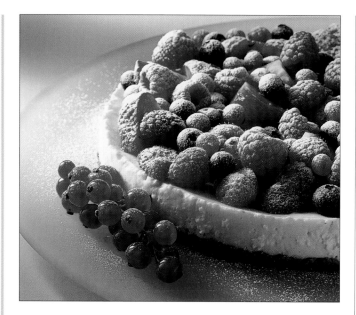

LEMON BERRY CHEESECAKE

264 cals, 12 g fat per serving
Serves 8

Many dieters find cheesecake a terrible temptation. This reduced fat version, however, will not pile on the pounds and is packed with healthy summer fruits.

115 g/4 oz ginger snaps, crushed (about ¾ cup)
25 g/1 oz (2 tbsp) low-fat margarine, melted
grated zest and juice of 2 medium lemons (about ⅓ cup juice)
1 tbsp plus 1 tsp unflavored gelatine
500 g/16 oz nonfat cream cheese, softened
230 g/8 oz nonfat plain yogurt
½ cup skim milk
80 g/2½ oz (⅓ cup) granulated sugar
450 g/1 lb (about 4 cups) mixed berries, such as strawberries,
  blueberries, and raspberries
confectioners sugar for dusting

■ Preheat the oven to 160°C/325°F. With a fork, mix the crushed ginger snaps and melted margarine and press into the base of a 20-cm/8-in springform pan or flan pan with removable bottom. Bake for 10 minutes or until firm to the touch.
■ Place 3 tbsp of the lemon juice in a small heatproof bowl and sprinkle the gelatine over it. Let soften for 5 minutes, then place the bowl in a saucepan of barely simmering water and leave until the gelatine has completely dissolved.
■ In a food processor or the bowl of an electric mixer, blend the cream cheese, yogurt, milk, granulated sugar, and remaining lemon juice and zest until smooth. Pour in the gelatine mixture and quickly process to blend in.
■ Pour the mixture over the base, cover, and chill for at least 3 hours or until set.
■ To serve, arrange the berries over the crust and dust with the confectioners sugar.

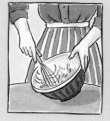

HEALTHY EATING TIP
Raspberries, strawberries, and cranberries contain ellagic acid, which may help prevent certain kinds of cancer. These fruits are also high in vitamin C, one of the better known antioxidants.

RASPBERRY ICE

125 cals, trace fat per serving
Serves 4

Strawberries can also be used for this dessert, which is an excellent low-calorie alternative to ice cream.

⅓ cup lime juice
115 g/4 oz (½ cup) sugar
⅓ cup water
(450 g/16 oz) frozen dry pack raspberries, thawed
mint leaves for garnish

■ In a medium-size saucepan, bring the lime juice, sugar, and water to a boil over moderate heat. Cook for about 1 minute or until the sugar is dissolved.
■ In a food processor or blender, purée the raspberries. Press the fruit through a fine sieve to eliminate the seeds. You should have 1⅓ cups purée; if not, add a little water.
■ Stir the purée into the sugar syrup until well combined. Transfer the mixture to an 8-in square baking pan, cover with plastic food wrap, and freeze for 2 hours or until the center is almost frozen. Remove the sorbet from the freezer, transfer to a large mixing bowl, and beat with an electric mixer until smooth. Return to the freezer for 45 minutes, then beat again until smooth. Freeze 2 to 3 hours more or until firm.
■ To serve, divide equally among four footed glass dishes or dessert bowls. Garnish with the mint leaves.

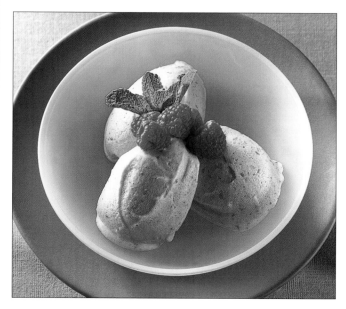

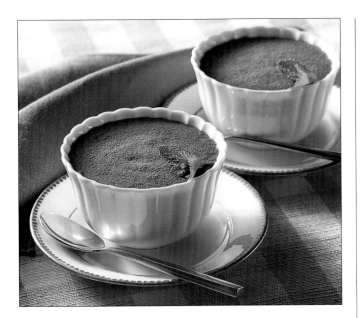

CHOCOLATE CREAM

84 cals, 0.5 g fat per serving

Serves 4

This creamy pudding will satisfy chocolate lovers without ruining their diet plans.

1 square (1 ounce) unsweetened chocolate
2 cups skim milk
⅓ cup granulated sugar
3 tbsp cornstarch
1 tsp vanilla extract

■ In the top half of a double boiler over simmering water, melt the chocolate. Stir in 1¾ cups of the milk and the sugar and continue stirring until the milk is very hot.

■ In a cup, blend the cornstarch with the remaining ¼ cup of milk; stir into the hot chocolate mixture. Cook, stirring constantly, until thickened and smooth. Cover and cook 15 minutes more, then stir in the vanilla.

■ Spoon the pudding into serving bowls, cover with plastic wrap, and chill for at least three hours.

DAILY MEAL PLAN

Breakfast: Menu 3 (page 132)
Mid-morning snack: 20 g/¾ oz blueberries with 100 g/3½ oz low-fat yogurt
Lunch: Curried Chicken Pitas (page 141) with fresh salad and 2 slices of whole-wheat bread; mineral water
Dinner: Country Casserole (page 145) with boiled carrots and 2 whole-grain rolls; glass of fresh fruit juice
Dessert: Chocolate Cream; herbal tea

Total for the day: 1,468 calories, 26 g fat

BAKED STUFFED APPLES WITH CUSTARD

270 cals, 0.5 g fat per serving

Serves 4

The high fructose content of apples helps to control blood sugar levels and the vitamin C content boosts the immune system. Custard is an ideal accompaniment, adding protein and calcium.

4 Rome beauty or other baking apples, about 225 g/8 oz each
115 g/4 oz (¾ cup) raisins
8 whole cloves
60 ml/¼ cup water

For the custard:
480 ml/ (2 cups) skim milk
40 g/3 tbsp granulated sugar
2 tbsp cornstarch

■ Preheat the oven to 190°C/375°F. Wash the apples well and remove the cores with an apple corer. Make a shallow cut through the skin around the middle of each apple. Stand them in an ovenproof dish in which they fit tightly enough to stay upright during cooking.

■ Stuff the center of each apple with the raisins and push two cloves into the skin. Pour the water into the bottom of the dish. Bake for about 30 minutes or until the apples are cooked through.

■ To make the custard, in a cup or small bowl, blend 2 tbsp of the milk with the cornstarch until it forms a smooth paste. In a medium-size saucepan, stir together the remaining milk, the sugar, and the milk-cornstarch mixture and bring to a boil, stirring until the custard thickens. Serve the apples warm or cold with a few spoonfuls of custard spooned over each one.

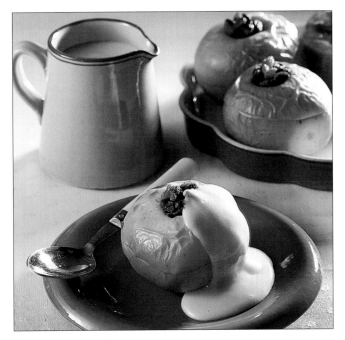

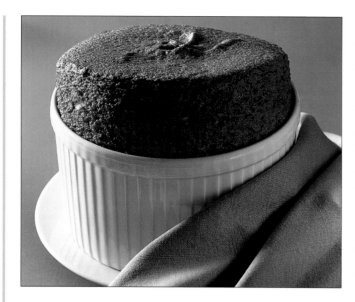

CURRANT SOUFFLÉ

92 cals, trace fat per serving

Serves 4

This handsome dessert is strong on flavor and rich in vitamin C. If currants are unavailable, substitute any flavorsome fruit such as raspberries or blueberries.

450 g/1 lb currants, blueberries, or other berries in season
55 g/2 oz (¼ cup) granulated sugar
4 egg whites, whipped until stiff peaks form

■ Preheat the oven to 190°C/375°F. Wash the currants, remove any stems, and put in a medium saucepan. Add the sugar and a little water and bring to a boil. Lower the heat and simmer, stirring occasionally, for 15 to 20 minutes.
■ Sieve the fruit or blend in a food processor until it is thick and smooth. It should make about 300 ml/1¼ cups purée.
■ Carefully fold the purée into the egg whites so that they are well mixed yet all the air is retained.
■ Transfer the mixture to a lightly greased 18 cm/7-in soufflé dish and bake for 25 minutes until it is well risen and brown on top. Serve immediately.

DAILY MEAL PLAN

BREAKFAST: *Menu 4 (page 132)*
MID-MORNING SNACK: *Peach*
LUNCH: *Mediterranean Tomato Soup (page 135) with 2 whole-wheat rolls; glass of mineral water*
DINNER: *Fish Kebabs, Ratatouille (page 146), and 150 g/5 oz boiled potatoes; glass of fruit juice*
DESSERT: *Currant Soufflé; cup of herbal tea or glass of mineral water*

TOTAL FOR THE DAY: *1,208 calories, 25.5 g fat*

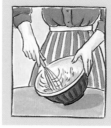

HEALTHY EATING TIP

One egg white contains only 16 calories and none of the fat and cholesterol found in egg yolks. When beaten, it makes a light, ideal addition to desserts for weight conscious people.

COEUR À LA CRÈME

155 cals, 4 g fat per serving

Serves 4

The fat-reduced dairy products on supermarket shelves today allow the full nutritional benefits of dairy foods to be enjoyed without too many calories. Dairy foods are rich in protein, calcium, and vitamin B$_{12}$.

340 g/12 oz cottage cheese, sieved or puréed until smooth
150 g/5½ oz (⅔ cup) low-fat plain yogurt
juice of half a lemon
2 tsp unflavored gelatine
6 apricots, peeled and pits removed
12 raspberries for garnish

■ In a bowl combine the cottage cheese, yogurt, and lemon juice. In a heatproof cup, soak the gelatine in 2 tbsp of cold water for 5 minutes. Place the cup in a pan of simmering water until the gelatine dissolves; stir into the cheese mixture.
■ Divide the cheese mixture among four heart-shaped moulds with a capacity of 100 ml/3½ fl oz and chill in the refrigerator for 24 hours.
■ In a food processor or blender, purée the apricots with 1 tbsp water until smooth. Carefully turn out the creams from the moulds onto individual plates; pour a little of the puréed fruit over each one, and garnish with the fresh raspberries.

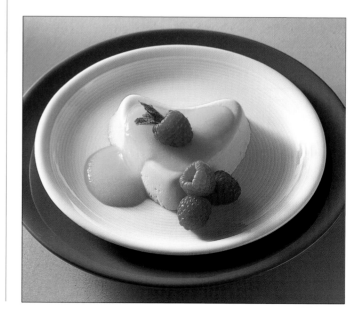

INDEX

ACKNOWLEDGMENTS

Carroll & Brown Limited
would like to thank
British Dietetics Association
British Food and Drink Federation
Penny Hunking, Energise, Surrey
Tessa Prior, Infant & Dietetics Food
    Association, London
The Pritikin Longevity Centre
Slimming World
Tesco Stores
Weight Watchers UK and Weight
    Watchers International, Inc,
    New York, USA
Wendy Doyle, Nutritionist

Editorial assistance
Richard Emerson
Sharon Freed
Simon Warmer

Design assistance
Simon Daley
Mari Hughes
Matt Sanderman

Photograph sources
  8 Rex Features/Tim Rooke
  9 Courtesy of The Pritikin
     Longevity Centre
 10 Image Bank/David De Lossy
 11 Popperfoto
 12 Science Photo Library/Prof. P.
     Motta/Dept. of anatomy/
     university 'La Sapienza', Rome
 16 National Gallery, London/
     Bridgeman Art Library, London
 17 (Top) Helsinki City Museum's
     Photographic Archive, (Bottom)
     Pictorial Press
 19 The National Trust Photo Library
 20 Zefa-Stockmarket
 22 Tony Stone Worldwide/David
     Madison

 29 Images Colour Library
 35 (Bottom) Tony Stone
     Images/Dennis O'Clair
 36 Science Photo Library/Oscar
     Burriel
 41 Courtesy of Professor Fairburn
 43 Corbis-Bettmann
 46 Hutchison Library/Lesley Melson
 47 Tony Stone Images/Philip &
     Karen Smith
 54 Images Colour Library
 58 Angela Hampton/Family Life
     Pictures
 61 Tony Stone Images/Jon Gray
 62 Tony Stone Images/Nick Dolding
 78 Tony Stone Images/David
     Madison
 85 John Walmsley
 88 Private Collection/Bridgeman Art
     Library, London
 92 Courtesy of the National College
     of Naturopathic Medicine,
     Portland, Oregon, US
 94 World View/Igno
     Cuypers/Science Photo Library
 95 Tony Stone Images/Christopher
     Bissell
 97 (Top) Explorer/JL Charmet,
     (Bottom) Wellcome Institute,
     London
 98 Novosti/Bridgeman Art Library,
     London
100 (Top) Pictorial Press Limited,
     (Bottom) The Hutchison
     Library/Errington
101 Tony Stone Images/Leland Bobbe
112 Tony Stone Images/Christopher
     Bissell
113 Russ Capps, photographer
114 Courtesy of Weight Watchers
     International, Inc
116 Tony Stone Images/Lori A. Peek
119 Tony Stone Images/Doug Armand

Medical illustrators
Sandie Hill
Paul Williams

Illustrators
Victor Ambrus
Janie Coath
Lorraine Harrison
Bill Piggins
Christine Pilsworth
Sarah Venus

Photographic assistants
M-A Hugo
Mark Langridge

Hair and make-up
Rachel Atwood
Bettina Graham
Kym Menzies

Picture researcher
Sandra Schneider

Food preparation
Maddalena Bastianelli
Eric Treuillé

Research
Steven Chong

Index
Steven Chong
Laura Price

Note
Metric and imperial measures are given throughout except when calculating
measures of nutrients, which are given in metric only. Calorie and fat contents
for foods and recipes are a guide only as it is not possible to give precise figures.